Advance Praise for *Choo*

In *Choose Better, Live Better*, Alan Carpenter goes way beyond the basics we know of living a healthy lifestyle, providing a roadmap to living a longer, more fruitful life. Through extensive research, and with great practical clarity, even the healthiest of us will better understand the keys to nurturing one's body, mind and spirit!
— Barry Siff, Former President USA Triathlon, Ultra Endurance Athlete

We can all use more energy, vitality, and better health, and we can all find simple effective advice for getting there in *Choose Better, Live Better*. Alan Carpenter's compelling narrative boils down a host of research into 9 "do-able" steps we can take, one at a time. No excuses—buy this book and take one step towards living better—your family, community, and healthcare system will thank you!
— Porter Storey MD, FACP, FAAHPM

Awakened by a close call after a mountaineering accident, Alan Carpenter realized that he had taken life for granted. Since then, he has set out to rejuvenate his own life—and help others along the way. The result: *Choose Better, Live Better*. If you're looking for a straightforward, helpful book on how you can improve your life through daily choices, this book is a terrific find. In user-friendly language, Carpenter summarizes the research on the benefits of lifestyle changes, such as moving more, eating better and living with purpose—and then provides practical ways to get started. No matter where you are on your path to better health, I recommend it!
— Laura Putnam, Author of *Workplace Wellness That Works* and CEO & Founder of Motion Infusion

A really well-done book with a wonderful message: What you do away from the table is just as important as what you eat! Highly recommended.
— Jonny Bowden, PhD, CNS aka "The Nutrition Myth Buster™", best-selling author of *The Great Cholesterol Myth, Living Low Carb, and The 150 Healthiest Foods on Earth*

Health is a choice—a conscious decision you can make. More, vitality is a choice—to remain vital and vibrant. Alan Carpenter lays out the path for you to have a lifetime of vitality. Now it's your decision.
— Will Murray, author of *The Four Pillars of Triathlon: Vital Mental Conditioning for Endurance Athletes*

In his fascinating new book, Alan Carpenter explores nine lifestyle choices which nurture body, mind, and spirit. The benefits of these lifestyle choices are backed by clinical research, but Carpenter also practices them himself, so he writes from the perspective of personal experience. Best of all, Carpenter explains how to turn healthy choices into long-term habits, which is the secret sauce of lifelong well-being. As someone who has practiced these habits for more than a decade, I am grateful for good health and a joyful life. If you want to enjoy better health, read this book and put its principles into action!

— Thomas Cross, Pastor, Broomfield United Methodist Church

Humans comprise a body, mind, and spirit. But more often than not, the medical establishment and books on healthy living ignore or gives short shrift to the spiritual aspects of human existence. *Choose Better, Live Better* addresses the full range of the human experience. Read this book to learn the surprising extent to which spiritually-related lifestyle choices predict better health and well-being.

— Harold Koenig, MD, Director, Center for Spirituality, Theology and Health, Duke University Medical Center

Alan Carpenter's book helped me to expand my knowledge of the patient's "Biopsychosocial Model" of their own health continuum. I appreciate his approach to wellness, and can see that this book will benefit people of all ages and health conditions. I will be keeping a copy of his book on my office shelf to share with my patients!

— William H. Dodson, III, MD, Family Physician Boulder, CO

Standing out in a crowded field of books related to life choices can be challenging. However, Alan's deep, research-based content, personalized with his powerful and authentic experiences, makes *Choose Better, Live Better* a clear leader for those looking to create lifelong health and well-being. Alan's nine lifestyle choices are practical, achievable, and results-oriented. He brings them to life through anecdotes, scientific research, and effective "to-do" lists. Feeling out of sorts? Feeling low energy? Feeling depleted or that your life could have more meaning, more joy, more well-being? Get this book—today.

— Robert Tipton, Author of *JUMP! - Get Unstuck,
Extraordinary Life Breakthroughs*

HOW TO CREATE LIFELONG HEALTH & WELL-BEING
Nine Lifestyle Choices That Nurture Body, Mind & Spirit

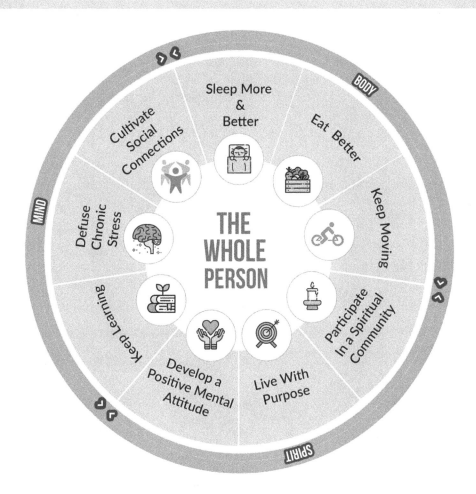

Alan T. Carpenter, PhD

CHOOSE BETTER, LIVE BETTER

Nine Healthy Choices that Nurture Body, Mind, and Spirit

Alan T Carpenter, PhD

Healthy Living Resources

Choose Better, Live Better
Nine Healthy Choices that Nurture Body, Mind, and Spirit
by Alan T Carpenter, PhD

Published by
Healthy Living Resources
2941 20th Street
Boulder, CO 80304

ISBN: 978-1-7342544-0-2
LCCN: 2020901990

Book Design: Nick Zelinger, www.NZGraphics.com
Editors: Jody Berman, www.BermanEditorial.com
        Janine Gastineau, www.JanineGastineau.com

Books may be purchased in quantity by contacting the publisher directly:
alantcarpenter@comcast.net

First Edition

10 9 8 7 6 5 4 3 2 1

1. Health   2. Well-being   3. Body, Mind, Spirit   4. Holistic Health

Printed in the United States

I dedicate this book to those intrepid individuals who want to take their lives to a higher level of consciousness.

Contents

Introduction

Out of the thousands of billing codes for thousands of medical services, there is not a single one for "wellness," or keeping patients in good health, which of course is the ultimate goal of every doctor and nurse and participant.
—George Halvorson[1]

Americans spend 92 cents of every medical care dollar on diagnosing and treating illnesses and diseases, and only 8 cents on preventing them[2]. Yet, according to the Centers for Disease Control and Prevention, preventable chronic diseases account for 75 percent of U.S medical care spending[3] (CDCP). Moreover, the surge in chronic diseases, including type 2 diabetes and obesity, threatens the ability of our medical system to cope effectively with an increased demand for treatment[4].

> More than 70 percent of Americans over age 65 exhibit two or more chronic diseases. Plus the growth of the U.S. population age 65 and older exceeds that of the rest of the U.S. population[5]. Yet, the Division of Aging Biology of the U.S. National Institute on Aging receives less than one percent of the total National Institutes of Health budget[6].

The advancing age of baby boomers, combined with progress in medicine and technology, will lead to an explosion in the number of Americans living to age 80 and beyond[7]. Aging baby boomers will almost certainly increase demands on America's medical system—demands that could become overwhelming. Half of today's 70-year-old boomers are projected to live to age 85. Three million of those folks are projected have Alzheimer's. (And that's not counting boomers who need medical care for other chronic conditions, such as type 2 diabetes or disability.) The prevalence of Alzheimer's disease and other dementias is expected to double by 2050[8]. For the year 2010, the estimated $109 billion price tag of dementia care purchased in the marketplace exceeded the comparable medical care costs of heart disease ($102 billion) and cancer ($77 billion)!

As if this weren't enough, we as a nation, and older people in particular, face the double-edged sword of reduced income to pay for medical care, plus reduced governmental revenues to fund Medicare and Medicaid due to projected national declines in payroll taxes. And what about older people who lose their mobility and can't care for themselves?

Our medical care system may be headed for disaster. Medical care expenses in the U.S. are increasing at an alarming rate, much faster than the overall rate of inflation[9]. While the stratospheric rise in the cost of health care plans has abated over the past few years, annual increases in health care plan costs are double those of inflation. Our current model of medical care is not financially sustainable. Making healthy choices and turning them into habits has the potential to reduce this looming financial problem and, in the process, substantially ease human suffering[10].

A Better Way Forward: Healthy Lifestyle Choices

Contrary to popular belief, better health and well-being don't typically depend on our genes, better medical care, or good luck. The single greatest opportunity to improve health and reduce premature deaths in the U.S. arises when we make healthy lifestyle choices[11]. In other words, choose better, live better.

Cancer researchers at the University of Texas proposed that our genes explain just 5–10 percent of most chronic illnesses, with lifestyle and environment accounting for the rest. More specifically, the researchers argued that cancer is largely preventable, *if we adopt* major lifestyle changes. Thus, adopting healthy lifestyle choices can tip the scale strongly in favor of our avoiding chronic diseases, including cancer, and achieving lifelong vibrant health and well-being[12].

Nearly half (!) of the deaths in our country eventually result from the daily choices we make. To paraphrase William Shakespeare, the trouble, dear reader, lies not in the stars, but in ourselves. We often make poor, largely unconscious decisions that lead to decay rather than vibrant health and well-being.

According to a 2004 report in the *Journal of the American Medical Association*, nine lifestyle factors, all of which we can control, accounted for 48 percent of U.S. deaths in year 2000. Tobacco, poor diet, inactivity, and excessive alcohol consumption caused 38 percent of those deaths. In fact, poor diet and inactivity may soon overtake smoking as *the leading causes of death in the U.S.*[14].

The good news: We have the power to make better choices every day. In doing so, we can stack the deck in favor of lifelong health and well-being by preventing—or at

Genes and Our Health

Our genes do not control our health to the degree and in the manner that many of us assume. Studies of identical twins raised apart can distinguish the influences of genetics from all other factors. For example, a 1996 study of 2,872 Danish twin pairs showed that only 25 percent of their longevity arose from their genetic makeup[13]. The other 75 percent reflected the daily choices they made and environmental influences.

By and large, genes do not predetermine our future. Rather, our genes create a template of possibilities. The way we conduct our lives (including what we eat and how much we move, among other things) and the environment in which we live affects the expression of our genes. While we may inherit a gene that predisposes us to breast cancer, the expression of that gene isn't a foregone conclusion. How we live is generally far more important than the existence of a harmful gene.

least postponing—chronic diseases and increasing the likelihood that illness and disability (if they happen at all) won't occur until our final few years of life. We'll live better while we're living longer, thereby extending what I call our *Quality of Lifespan*—the number of years of life during which we function at a high level. Thus, our *Quality of Lifespan* increases as our longevity increases and as we maintain high functionality. Embracing the nine healthy lifestyle choices can increase our *Quality of Lifespan*.

Nine Healthy Lifestyle Choices That Nurture Body, Mind, and Spirit

This book presents nine easy-to-understand, practical, evidence-based healthy lifestyle choices that nurture body, mind, and spirit (see chart). Embracing these nine lifestyle choices provides a comprehensive approach that encompasses our entire being, not just our physical body. In my view, the triad of body, mind, and spirit captures the breadth of human existence. (Medical practitioners typically ignore the spiritual dimension of the human experience.) Embracing these healthy lifestyle choices can improve our health, elevate our well-being, and prevent or at least postpone many if not all chronic diseases. The following chart summarizes the nine healthy lifestyle choices and some of the benefits that we can expect from following them.

A Word on Well-Being

As noted on the following page, the nine lifestyle choices nurture more than our physical health. These lifestyle choices also enhance our overall well-being. In 2004, prominent psychologists Ed Diener and Martin Seligman defined well-being as "peoples' positive evaluations of their lives, including positive emotion, engagement, satisfaction, and meaning." Diener and Seligman identified a number of benefits of

Nine Healthy Lifestyle Choices

Three healthy choices that nurture our **Body:**

1. *Keep Moving.* Whole-body movement, like walking, builds the physical and mental capability to operate effectively in the world.
2. *Eat Better.* High-quality food provides the energy and nutrients to live each day to the fullest.
3. *Sleep More and Better.* Sufficient restful sleep yields a daily physical and mental recharge.

Three healthy choices that nurture our **Mind:**

1. *Cultivate Social Connections.* Maintaining social relationships creates a sense of mutual caring and connectedness to others.
2. *Defuse Chronic Stress.* Developing effective ways to respond to life's demands reduces our body's stress response and builds peace of mind.
3. *Keep Learning.* Using our brain, especially in novel ways, maintains or potentially increases neural connections that keep our mind sharp, durable, and creative.

Three healthy choices that nurture our **Spirit:**

1. *Develop a Positive Mental Attitude.* Embracing life with optimism, forgiveness, and gratitude can improve our emotional well-being.
2. *Live with Purpose.* Finding ways to live purposefully and serve others can create a meaningful life.
3. *Participate in a Spiritual Community.* Being part of a spiritual community can help us manifest our Higher Self in the world.

well-being: (1) more effective functioning at work and at home, (2) better social relationships, (3) higher productivity at work, (4) higher incomes, and (5) better mental and physical health[15]. Following a lengthy literature review, Diener and Seligman concluded that high well-being arises from the following: (1) a stable democratic society that provides at least the basic material resources, (2) supportive friends and family, (3) rewarding and engaging work and adequate income, (4) reasonable health and accessible treatment for mental problems, (5) important goals related to one's values, and (6) a philosophy or religion that provides guidance, purpose, and meaning in life. Diener and Seligman lamented that Americans don't have "ready and concrete models of how to pursue the goal of well-being." The book you're holding today attempts to provide such a model. Adopting the nine healthy lifestyle choices can increase your well-being.

The Power of Healthy Lifestyle Choices

Many people think that the effects of their daily choices on health and well-being pale in comparison to the miracles of modern medications, surgical procedures, and medical devices. *Modern medicine can often control the symptoms of chronic diseases but cannot cure—much less prevent—them.* Research shows that our daily choices typically determine how far we will progress on the path to lifelong health and well-being. That's empowering. We have the power to create lifelong health and well-being through the daily choices we make. Consider the following:

Dr. Walter Willett at Harvard is one of the most widely published experts on the health effects of the foods people eat. He estimates that eating a Mediterranean-type diet (whole grains/cereals, fruits/vegetables, beans, nuts, fish, olive oil, wine, limited red meat), along with engaging in regular physical activity and not smoking, can reduce our risk of type 2 diabetes by 90 percent, coronary heart disease by 80 percent, and stroke by 70 percent! Imagine what could happen if we were to embrace these and other healthy choices, such as *Sleep More and Better, Cultivate Social Connections, and Develop a Positive Mental Attitude.* Our risk of dying from coronary heart disease would likely drop even further and/or be postponed until much later in life. Our risk of type 2 diabetes might drop to near zero[16].

In 1980, James Fries, a doctor and researcher at Stanford University, proposed that people who take care of themselves by making healthy choices would not only live longer but also live better, staving off chronic illness, cognitive decline, and debilitative accidents. He predicted that most of the illness or injury that does occur would be compressed into the last few years of life. Studies by Fries and others support this proposition, which he called the 'compression of morbidity hypothesis.' Fries and his colleagues studied male and female members of a running club in California. Disability of the runners increased but only between ages 75 and 79. The runners experienced significantly lower mortality than the non-runners, resulting in an estimated two years of extra longevity for the former. Keep Moving was a key aspect of prolonging both a longer and a disability-free life[17].

Fries and colleagues also found that survivors in the healthy choices group (moderate body-mass index, no smoking, near-daily exercise) had half the disability risk and postponed the onset of disability for about five years, compared to survivors in the unhealthy choices group. Therefore, making healthy choices can increase our *Quality of Lifespan*[18].

Healthy Choices and a Self-Actualized Life

The famed psychologist Abraham Maslow developed the hierarchy of needs in his 1954 book, *Motivation and Personality*. The nine healthy choices presented in this book map well on Maslow's hierarchy[19].

Maslow's Hierarchy of Needs and the Nine Healthy Lifestyle Choices	
Level 1: Physiological	*Keep Moving, Eat Better, Sleep More and Better, Defuse Chronic Stress*
Level 2: Safety	*Cultivate Social Connections*
Level 3: Belonging	*Cultivate Social Connections*
Level 4: Esteem	*Develop a Positive Mental Attitude, Keep Learning*
Level 5: Self-Actualization	*Live with Purpose, Participate in a Spiritual Community*

The Benefits of Making Healthy Choices Early in Life

Chronic conditions, like cardiovascular disease, account for a high percentage of illnesses and deaths in the U.S. Preventive measures largely target adults; however, some chronic conditions appear to have their roots in childhood[20]. Thus, adopting healthy choices early in life will likely reduce our risk of developing a chronic disease in adulthood.

Dr. Henry McGill at the University of Texas Health Science Center at San Antonio believes that *90 percent of heart attacks are preventable.* A key aspect of reducing the lifetime risk of heart attack is beginning preventive measures early in life. Cardiovascular disease is a chronic condition that can start early in life. In one study, the prevalence of coronary artery lesions rose dramatically from adolescence to ages 30–39. The risk of advanced coronary artery lesions dropped progressively as the number of healthy lifestyle choices increased, indicating that healthy lifestyle choices early in life might cause fewer lesions[21].

Coronary artery calcification occurs early in the process of coronary artery plaque development, which leads to cardiovascular disease. People who scored higher on a global hostility scale had a nearly 10-fold higher risk of coronary artery calcification compared to those who scored lower on hostility. Therefore, it appears that young adults who also reduce their aggression, anger, and resentment might greatly reduce their risk of cardiovascular disease[22].

What about aerobic fitness early in life? Evidently, intensive aerobic training during young adulthood can translate into greater aerobic fitness much later in life. In 1968, twenty-six male runners training for the 1968 Olympics also participated in an aerobic fitness study. In 2013, researchers revisited these athletes, measuring heart rate, VO_2 max (a measure of the maximum rate of oxygen consumption), ventilation, and running economy for 22 of them (three had died, one declined to participate). The results showed that higher fitness in 1968 contributed to higher-than-expected fitness 45 years later. Aerobic fitness created earlier in life persisted at relatively high levels over more than four decades[23].

Biological aging can begin relatively early in life. Researchers recently estimated the rate of biological aging for 954 individuals born in 1972–1973 in Dunedin, New Zealand, and followed from birth to age 38. Data for 18 biomarkers (such as cardiorespiratory fitness, waist-to-hip ratio, triglycerides) were collected for all participants at ages 26, 32, and 38. Researchers calculated each individual's "pace of aging" using data for the 18 biomarkers. The results showed that biological aging was well underway at age 38, with the biological age of many individuals registering as greater than their chronological age. Individuals with a more rapid pace of aging showed diminished objective measures of physical capability and cognitive functioning and had worse artery and vein health than those with a slower pace of aging. Finally, those with a greater pace of aging were judged to be older, based on a picture of each face, than those with a slower pace of aging. The bottom line: if we make healthy choices early on and turn these choices into habits, we can reap major benefits over the long term[24].

"Act now like you will need your body for a hundred years."
—Karl Pillemer[25], *30 Lessons for Living*

It's Never Too Late to Begin Making Healthy Choices

Even at an advanced age, making healthy choices can improve our strength and well-being. A classic study by Maria Fiatarone and colleagues published in 1990 made this point convincingly. Muscle weakness and accompanying mobility impairment in elderly persons increase their risk of falls, fractures, and dependency on others for activities of daily life. Frail nursing home residents ranging in age from 86 to 96 participated in eight weeks of high-intensity strength training. They made dramatic gains in muscle strength and size and functional mobility. For example, quadriceps muscle strength (the average of both legs) increased by 176 percent. The results are particularly impressive given participants' advanced age, sedentary lifestyle, multiple chronic conditions, functional disabilities, and nutritional inadequacies [26].

Researchers investigated the link between diet and lifestyle factors for older European men and women with an average age of 73 and 77, respectively. The low-risk group was defined as adhering to four healthy lifestyle factors: (1) following a modified Mediterranean diet; (2) drinking moderate amounts of alcohol; (3) never smoking or quitting more than 15 years prior to the study; and (4) physical activity in the top one-third of participants. Compared to other participants, older folks with all four healthy life-style factors reduced their risk of all-cause mortality by more than 50 percent over 10 years[27]. Wow!

Still not convinced that healthy choices matter much? A study of 17,989 generally healthy Medicare-eligible patients at the Cooper Clinic in Dallas showed that higher midlife cardiorespiratory fitness was associated with a 16 percent lower risk of depression. After a diagnosis of depression, achieving higher levels of fitness at midlife was associated with a 56 percent lower risk of cardiovascular mortality. Those in the highest quintile of fitness had a higher risk of dying than developing a chronic disease. This means that chronic conditions that did occur happened *later in life*. These results support James Fries' "compression of morbidity" hypothesis—namely, that healthy lifestyle choices (especially *Keep Moving*) can reduce or eliminate the risk of chronic conditions (a.k.a. morbidity) and disability until the last few years of life[28].

Turn Healthy Choices into Habits

Once we make a healthy choice, the next step is to turn that choice into a habit. The automatic nature of a habit allows us to make a healthy choice with little or no conscious thought. We can save our willpower for other challenging situations. The more of these healthy habits we can create, the greater the benefits we will realize. We can expect more energy, better brain function, and greater happiness, among many positive outcomes. Plus, these habits will likely reduce our risk of numerous chronic conditions, including cardiovascular disease, stroke, and Alzheimer's disease. People who make one healthy choice and turn it into a habit often find themselves making additional healthy choices without consciously deciding to do so.

Making Healthy Choices for Healthy Aging

Most Americans don't make many of the nine healthy lifestyle choices. Nevertheless, if you were to ask 100 people whether physical exercise is beneficial, 99 would probably say yes. In spite of this widespread belief, only 19 percent of women, 20 percent of adolescents, and 26 percent of men in America meet the federal recommendations for physical activity (150 minutes per week at moderate intensity), according to the 2018 Physical Activity Guidelines for Americans published by the U.S. Department of Health and Human Services[31].

Because the aging of the U.S. population has potentially catastrophic consequences for the American medical health care system, translating research findings about "healthy aging" into tangible, beneficial results should be a top priority for public health authorities. For example, research supports the importance of *Cultivate Social Connections* with respect to later-life health and well-being, including greater longevity, greater cognitive function, lower risk of depression, less risk of falling, and the greater ability to maintain activities of daily living[32]. Research also

A Lesson from the Old Order Amish

A study in 1981 showed that Old Order Amish men had lower mortality rates than non-Amish Caucasian men, in spite of the fact that Amish men made much less use of modern medical care[29]. A more recent study extended this line of research.

This time, the comparison population for the Old Order Amish (both men and women) included participants in the Framingham Heart Study (residents of Framingham, MA) with comparable birth dates who also survived to at least age 30. The Amish men lived an estimated three years longer than non-Amish men.

More striking, the rate of hospitalization was far lower for Amish men and women in 16 out of 18 diagnostic categories. Amish women had a higher rate of hospital admissions for complications of pregnancy, but that difference arose largely from them giving birth to an average of seven children. Amish men had a higher rate of shows that *Keep Moving* is one of the strongest predictors of multiple aspects of health and functioning in later life. There is little doubt that adopting these two healthy choices—not to mention the other seven—can increase our *Quality of Lifespan*. Will we Americans succeed in widely adopting healthy lifestyle choices such that healthy aging will become the new normal?

My Story

In 2008, I hiked the entire 218-mile-long John Muir Trail through the Sierra Nevada Mountains in California. That marvelous experience hooked me on long-distance hiking. During the following winter, my enthusiasm for hiking reached a point of irrational exuberance. I vowed to hike the entire 2,660-mile Pacific Crest Trail (PCT) from Mexico to Canada through California, Oregon, and Washington in one season. But life got in the way, and I kept postponing my PCT hike. Over the ensuing four years, I repeated my John Muir Trail hike and hiked the 486-mile Colorado Trail twice. Finally, on April 20, 2013, I set forth from the southern terminus of the Pacific Crest Trail, starting at the U.S.–Mexico border southeast of San

hospitalization for the category "symptoms, signs, and ill-defined conditions."

The study authors speculated that the Old Order Amish adopted lifestyle factors such as regular physical exercise, social support, and minimal cigarette smoking that led to better health, reduced hospitalizations, and greater longevity[30].

Adopting healthy lifestyle choices might produce better health outcomes for the rest of us at lower cost than improved medical technology and greater access to hospital care.

Diego. For the next 58 days, I hiked mostly alone through the semi-arid chaparral shrublands and deserts of Southern California, then through the Sierra Nevada Mountains, before hiking into the Cascade Range in central California. After covering 1,060 miles, I was living the dream. But not for long.

On June 16 (ironically, Father's Day), I rounded the steep north face of Mount Raymond in the Mokulumne Wilderness and stopped. A 20-foot-long sheet of hard, smooth ice covered the trail. Ravenous hunger gnawed at me. The prospect of stuffing my face at the all-you-can eat buffet at Harrah's Casino in South Lake Tahoe, a mere 33 miles up the trail, pulled me forward like a zombie. I started walking across the icy trail but slipped and hurtled 100 feet down a steep gully and slammed into a boulder.

After I regained consciousness, I made a life decision: I am going to survive. I made a simple plan. Stop the flow of blood gushing from a golf ball–sized hole in my leg. Then crawl out of the icy gulley then inch up the steep, rock-strewn mountainside back to the trail. Somehow, in spite of my injuries, overwhelming pain, and loose rocks, I managed to crawl back up to the trail. Somehow I managed to get a cell phone connection. Somehow Joe and Matt from the California Highway Patrol and their helicopter managed to pluck me from the mountainside and ferry me to a hospital in Reno, Nevada. I spent five days in the hospital being treated for fractured ribs, a partially collapsed lung, plus lots of cuts, scrapes, and bruises.

My wife Betsy flew to Reno and drove me back to our home in Boulder, Colorado. After a period of whining, complaining, and feeling sorry for myself, I had an epiphany. In my incapacitated condition, I realized that I'd taken my life for granted. I also realized how essential being active was to my life. I vowed to rejuvenate my life, but I wasn't sure how to do it. So I started to read while sitting on the sofa recovering at home. I read book after book about health and well-being. Before long, I discovered that my health and well-being were largely a matter of my own choosing. I kept reading, expanding my repertoire to include original scientific and medical research articles.

Over the past five-plus years, I've synthesized what I learned into the nine healthy lifestyle choices presented in this book. Scientific research and clinical experience support the efficacy of these choices. As I synthesized my research, I applied what I learned in my everyday life. I also field-tested these healthy lifestyle choices under demanding physical, mental, and spiritual conditions during subsequent long-distance hiking and cycling adventures. Since my accident at age 66, I have hiked and cycled over 12,000 miles on the Pacific Crest Trail, the Appalachian Trail, the Continental Divide Trail, and the Southern and Northern Tier bike routes, I expect to continue my long-distance adventures indefinitely.

This book presents evidence from over 500 published research studies. It provides a sampling of relevant research articles, but is not a thorough review of a voluminous literature. Nevertheless, I am confident that the studies referenced in the book constitute a fair representation of the relevant published studies.

How This Book Is Organized

This book has four parts. Part 1 discusses three healthy choices that nurture the body. Part 2 looks at three healthy choices that both nurture the mind and promote emotional, psychological, and social wellness. Part 3 covers three healthy choices that nurture the spirit and further support well-being. Each of the chapters in Parts 1–3 ends with a list of practical ways—action steps—to help you embrace the healthy lifestyle choice discussed in that chapter. You'll also find three key points that summarize that particular lifestyle choice. Reflecting upon these points can help you embed them firmly into your being. Your subconscious mind will then begin to alert you to opportunities in your life that will help you embrace that lifestyle choice.

The healthy choices discussed in Parts 1–3 typically focus on the benefits of embracing one healthy choice. But life really isn't a matter of making one healthy choice, at least not over the long haul. Part 4 highlights research showing the huge potential benefits of making multiple healthy lifestyle choices.

A short summary recaps the salient points covered in the book and suggests making healthy lifestyle choices one at a time. The Recommended Resources section includes books that I have found particularly useful in understanding the power of making healthy lifestyle choices. An even shorter appendix helps readers interpret the research studies highlighted in the book. The End Notes contains the literature citations for all the studies mentioned in the text.

* * *

Perhaps you've had a wake-up call in your life—like the accident I experienced—that created powerful motivation for you to make major life changes. Maybe you have at least one emotionally charged, overwhelmingly important reason—what I call a BIG WHY—to make healthy choices and enjoy the benefits they provide as a key part of your life. Whatever your reason, this book can help you begin immediately to move along the path of lifelong vibrant health and emotional well-being. Let's get started!

Part 1

Nurture Your Body with Three Healthy Choices

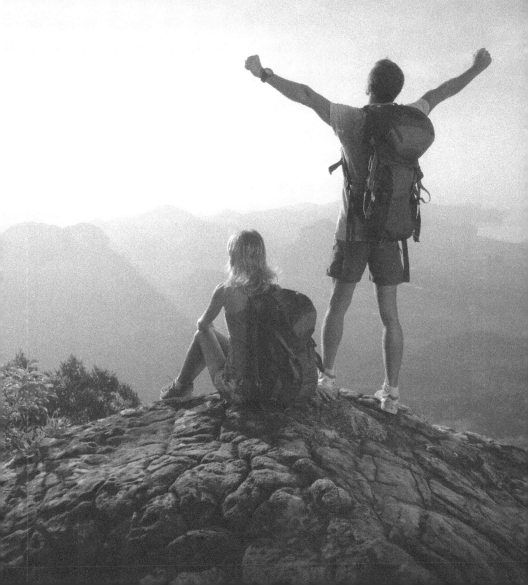

Chapter 1

Keep Moving

Fortunately, even quite late in life, an increase in physical activity is richly rewarded with health benefits.
—Gregory D. Cartee and colleagues[1]

Keep Moving may be the most important lifestyle choice of all. According to the MacArthur Foundation Study of Successful Aging, exercise is the crux of successful aging[2]. *Keep Moving* includes any type of whole-body movement, and the intensity of movement can vary widely. Generally, more strenuous movement produces greater benefits and faster results. *Keep Moving* also refers to interrupting an hour or more of sitting with short movement breaks.

Evolutionary Basis to *Keep Moving*

Humans evolved to move, walking perhaps 6-8 miles on a typical day in Paleolithic times[3]. Our forbearers moved much more and sat far less than the vast majority of contemporary Americans. Many scientists believe that human biochemical processes today closely reflect those of ancient pre-humans. Therefore, from an evolutionary perspective, it makes sense for our bodies to interpret being sedentary as a signal that life may end soon. Inactivity, especially in older people, signals decay.

We Americans move far less than our counterparts did just 60 years ago. Then most jobs involved manufacturing and required at least a moderate amount of physical energy. Today, most American jobs occur in the service and information sectors and are largely sedentary. One study showed that the energy expended at work from 1960-1962 to 2003-2006 declined by 142 calories per day for men. The reduction in energy expended over that period predicted an increase in body weight of adult men to 197 pounds, which closely matched the actual weight of 202 pounds. Actual weight gain for women also mirrored the predicted gain[4].

The same shift from being active to being sedentary at work also occurred in the home and in getting to and from work as Americans adopted more labor-saving devices. A study of Mayo Clinic employees showed that they burned 111 fewer calories a day by driving to work rather than walking, machine-washing dishes and clothes rather than hand-washing them, and using the elevator at work or in the apartment rather than climbing the stairs. Coincidentally, those who walked 45 minutes to work at two miles per hour expended about 111 calories of energy daily. Thus, trading an hour of sedentary time for 45 minutes of brisk walking would compensate for the reduced energy expenditure caused by using labor-saving devices at home[5].

Human biology evolved to cope with frequent food shortages—not today's super-abundant, highly palatable food and a sedentary existence. *Shifting our energy balance from accumulation to neutral would involve only modest adjustments in our lives.* For example, a 155-pound person walking briskly (taking at least 10 steps in a six-second period) for one extra mile per day (about 2,000 steps over 15–20 minutes) would burn an additional 100 calories. That extra 15–20 minutes of moving around would nearly eliminate obesity in the U.S., assuming no increase in food consumption[6].

Only 22.9 percent of U.S. adults aged 18-64 get the minimum recommended weekly 150 minutes of moderate intensity exercise, or 75 minutes of strenuous exercise[7]. Yet *Keep Moving* provides enormous positive effects on our health and well-being–more than most people realize.

All Types of Movement Are Beneficial

Whether it be aerobic, strength building, flexibility, or balance exercise, each form of movement is vital for vibrant health.

- **Aerobic.** *Aerobic* literally means "with oxygen." Common aerobic exercises include walking, running, cycling, stair climbing, spinning, swimming, and dancing. Our circulatory system, including blood vessels that nourish the heart and brain, is our main beneficiary of aerobic exercise. *The sweet spot for aerobic exercise is roughly 30 minutes per day.*

- **Strength building.** Strength building increases muscle mass, which is especially important as we age and lose muscle cells. Strength building through lifting weights, physical labor, yoga, and others activities increases the size of muscle cells, thereby increasing muscle mass. Strength building also increases muscle tone and power. More muscle boosts our metabolism, helping us to burn more calories, which can help prevent weight gain and support weight loss. *Health authorities recommend two or three strength building sessions each week.*

- **Flexibility.** Flexibility exercises help maintain healthy joints and retain full range of motion. Better joint health leads to less pain and greater likelihood that we can take care of everyday tasks later in life. *I recommend incorporating flexibility exercises into your twice- or thrice weekly strength-building routine.*

- Balance exercises. Maintaining balance in our later years cuts our risk of falling and breaking a hip or leg, thereby reducing our chances of ending up in a nursing home. Falls that result in hip or leg fractures require an extended period of *convalescence*. *For seniors, I recommend practicing flexibility and balance exercises three or more days each week.*

Interrupt Inactivity with Movement

Americans age six and older spend a *lot* of time sitting—some 7.7 hours a day[8]. Accumulating evidence suggests that inactivity acts an independent risk factor for major health problems, including diabetes, cardiovascular disease, and more[9]. Moving more is desirable, but it won't negate the adverse effects of extended sitting. If we spend too much time sitting rather than moving, we lose aerobic capacity, bone density, muscle mass, and muscle tone. To achieve vibrant health and well-being, we need to *Keep Moving*—several minutes each hour—*and* sit less. Short periods of activity can offset the negative effects of long periods of inactivity.

Benefits of *Keep Moving*

The scientific and clinical evidence for the health benefits of movement is overwhelming and indisputable. This section discusses the profound and positive impacts of *Keep Moving* on our health and well-being.

Benefits of *Keep Moving*

- Increased *Quality of Lifespan*
- Increased energy
- More calories burned
- Better blood sugar control
- Improved brain health
- Better mood
- Better self-control
- Improved bone health
- Maintained mobility

Increased *Quality of Lifespan*

Our *Quality of Lifespan* is the length of time we maintain high functionality in our life. That is, if we live longer and function at a higher level during those years, we increase our *Quality of Lifespan*. This concept integrates numerous benefits in health and well-being, including fewer chronic diseases and accidents, reduced chronic stress, and greater mobility and longevity. Seeking to increase our *Quality of Lifespan* may help us develop specific, positive goals that reflect what we truly want in life rather than what we don't want. Positive goals are more likely to create internal motivation to make and habituate healthy choices than negative goals. People who identify quality of life as a major part of their personal vision tend to *Keep Moving* more than people who don't[10].

With all its health benefits, physical exercise would seem to improve *Quality of Lifespan*. Researchers in Oklahoma sought to determine if that is true. They divided 112 volunteers (average age of 70) who were free of either obvious cardiovascular and/or obstructive pulmonary disease into a high-exercise group and a low-exercise group. Volunteers in the high-exercise group (who performed moderate physical activities for at least one hour per week) scored significantly higher in eight categories of health-related quality of life than volunteers in the low-exercise group (who performed moderate physical activities for less than one hour per week). Even after accounting for effects of gender and hypertension, members of the high-exercise group still scored significantly higher in physical functioning, vitality, social functioning, and bodily pain endurance.

Multicomponent physical training—including muscle power training, balance, and gait retraining—can reduce the risk of falls for older people and increase *Quality of Lifespan*. But would training be effective for the oldest of the old? A randomized controlled trial examined the effects of multicomponent training on muscle power output, muscle mass, and muscle tissue thinning, the risk of falls, and functional outcomes in 24 frail nonagenarians (persons aged 90–99) The physical training group performed a twice-weekly, 12-week multicomponent exercise program composed of muscle power training (8–10 repetitions) and balance and gait retraining. Compared to the non-exercise control group, the physical training group required significantly less time to rise from a chair or get up and walk. This group also demonstrated improved balance, a reduced incidence of falls, enhanced muscle strength, and increased muscle thickness and weight. Members of the non-exercise control group had significantly lower strength and functional outcomes. Routine multicomponent exercise training increased *Quality of Lifespan*, even for nonagenarians[11].

Data pooled from six longitudinal studies in the National Cancer Institute Cohort Consortium looked at the benefits of exercise in subjects whose mean age at baseline was 61 years, and whose mean age at follow-up was 71. More exercise predicted more years of life.

For example, those exercising 56 minutes per day had a 39 percent lower risk of death and 3.8 extra years of life. The beneficial effects of exercise continued up to about 70 minutes per day. Beyond this activity level, the health benefits of additional exercise appeared to plateau. But even low amounts of exercise, such as 10 minutes per day, were associated with increased longevity. The more we *Keep Moving*, the longer and better we're likely to live[12].

Might seniors be past the point where exercise is beneficial? Researchers with the Honolulu Heart Program investigated this question. The Honolulu Heart Program began in 1965 and followed 707 nonsmoking retired men of Japanese ancestry aged 61–81 at baseline. At 12 years of follow-up, researchers found that 43 percent of the men who walked less than one mile per day died, while only 2 percent (!) of those who walked over two miles per day died. A man who walked more than two miles per day lived an average of five years longer than a man who walked less than one mile per day[13]. Other observational studies provide tantalizing suggestions that physical activity increases survival of women diagnosed with breast cancer. Compared to patients who reported walking at an average pace for one hour per week, women who walked at an average pace for 3-5 hours per week reduced their risk of breast cancer recurrence by 50 percent, comparable to the effectiveness of a leading drug for breast cancer patients—but without the high expense or side effects[14].

Longitudinal studies with humans and animal models suggest that vigorous and moderate physical exercise during midlife protects against Parkinson's disease. A new systematic review and meta-analysis found that persons in the highest quintiles of total and moderate/vigorous physical activity had 21 and 29 percent lower risks, respectively, of developing Parkinson's disease. The benefit arose either from moderate or vigorous physical activity. Each increase in 10 metabolic-equivalent task-hours of physical activity per week (about 30 minutes of moderate-intensity exercise per day) predicted a 10 percent risk reduction in Parkinson's disease in men but not in women[15]).

Given that exercise and physical fitness predict reduced risks of dementia and cognitive decline in the general population, physical activity may reduce the progression of mental deterioration in patients with Parkinson's disease, and also reduce the risk of nursing home placement due to mental and physical infirmity[16]. Given the profound physical and mental effects of Parkinson's disease on *Quality of Lifespan*, devoting a half hour per day to *Keep Moving* would be a terrific investment.

Increased energy

Ironically, moving gives us more, not less, energy. That's why competitive athletes train—in part, because training, with lots of movements of various kinds, gives athletes more energy in terms of endurance and strength.

I offer a personal example from my long-distance hiking experience. On April 20, 2013, I set forth on the 2,660-mile-long Pacific Crest Trail (PCT) from the US–Mexico border southeast of San Diego. My intention was to walk to Canada over the next four-plus months. I hiked north for 58 days covering 1,061 miles through arid Southern California, then through the Sierra Nevada Mountains. On Father's Day, June 16, I made a breathtakingly boneheaded attempt to cross a short section of icy trail on a steep mountainside. I slipped and hurtled 100 feet down a steep and icy gulley before slamming into a boulder. That ended my PCT hike for 2013 and began a lengthy period of recuperation, during which time I adopted better lifestyle choices.

I resumed my hike on July 1, 2014, near the spot where I fell, and walked 1,599 miles in 70 days through the rest of California, Oregon, and Washington. In 2013, I averaged 18.3 miles per day and 22.4 miles per day in 2014, an increase of 25 percent. Walking more miles per day in 2014 happened in spite of being a year older, having suffered a life-threatening accident the year before, and hiking through more physically and mentally challenging terrain. I attribute my greater daily mileage in 2014 to the increased energy I felt from making healthy choices during the year after my accident.

More calories burned

We all know people who seem to not gain weight no matter what they eat, while others seem to gain weight just by looking at food. People who don't gain weight while eating more tend to move around more after they eat, thereby burning those extra calories and preventing them from turning into fat. People who do gain weight after they eat bigger helpings don't move around afterwards, with those extra calories turning into fat[17].

What we do in our daily life can dramatically affect our total daily energy output. A person can consume an extra 56,000 calories over a two-month period (nearly an extra 1,000 calories per day!) and still not gain weight, providing they simply walk a lot more. Many short walks (more than 12 minutes on average) at low speed (less than 1.1 mile per hour) add up. Even small increases in movement while accomplishing daily tasks can collectively tip the balance from gaining weight to staying trim. This may not seem to make much difference, but research shows that it does[18]. At its most basic, the lesson is to get out of the chair and *Keep Moving*.

Better blood sugar control

After we eat a meal, our blood sugar spikes in an hour or two, then declines until the next meal. Post-meal blood sugar levels typically rise with age. Post-meal increases in blood sugar may contribute to impaired glucose tolerance (pre-diabetes) and subsequent type 2 diabetes in older people. Insulin and physical exercise both independently stimulate the transport of blood sugar into muscle cells, thereby reducing blood sugar levels. Researchers in Washington, D.C., investigated whether short periods of post-meal exercise might lower blood sugar spikes. They found that post-meal walking (three times daily) reduced average blood sugar over three-hour and 24-hour periods for inactive, nonsmoking people over age 60. Post-meal exercise significantly controlled blood glucose for three hours, while the other exercise protocols did not. Developing a simple habit of taking a 22-minute walk starting 30 minutes after finishing dinner could substantially improve our health and reduce the risk of type 2 diabetes[19].

Improved brain health

Abundant studies suggest that physical exercise promotes proper brain functioning[20]. Exercise is related to both improved cognitive function and brain plasticity. The scientific literature indicates that exercise—both aerobic and strength training—is an effective treatment for depression. Clinical trials reveal that physical activity may also decrease depressive symptoms and improve the quality of life for Alzheimer's disease patients. Additionally, limited evidence suggests that physical exercise improves quality of life, functional fitness, and activities of daily living, as well as reduces neurological symptoms of patients with Parkinson's disease[21].

Regular physical activity throughout the life span, especially in old age, predicts improved overall health and reduced risk of dementia and Alzheimer's disease. Longitudinal studies reveal links between physical activity and risk of dementia. The mechanism for such improvement is unclear but may be due to better cerebral blood flow. The authors of a 2016 review concluded that physical training, with aerobic, strength, and balance components, improved brain function. Better function manifested in increased executive function, greater attentional capacity, faster processing speed, and better memory[22].

Numerous studies support the idea that physical activity protects against dementia. But what about older people who already have white matter changes (nerve cell deterioration) in their brain, potentially affecting nerve cell function? As part of a larger study, 638 older people were examined at baseline and then annually for three years. The subjects were Europeans with an average age of 74 years, free of disability, and with some degree of white matter changes as determined with magnetic resonance imaging. Even with white matter changes, physical activity predicted a lower risk of cognitive impairment and vascular dementia by 36 percent and 58 percent, respectively[23]. This study alone ought to motivate us to become more physically active.

Better mood

In 1982, the Japanese Ministry of Agriculture, Forestry, and Fisheries coined the term *shinrin-yoko*. It refers to making contact with or taking in the atmosphere of a forest. In a recent study, such "forest bathing" was shown to promote relaxation. Male undergraduate students from a Japanese university spent time sitting (about 14 minutes) and/or walking (about 16 minutes) in a forest on one day and in an urban environment on an adjacent day. The students' mood after forest viewing or walking changed in a favorable direction—less tension/anxiety and less anger/hostility—compared to urban viewing or walking. Similarly, salivary cortisol (a measure of stress), pulse rate, systolic and diastolic blood pressure, and the ratio of sympathetic to parasympathetic nervous system activity (a lower ratio indicates less stress) were significantly lower after forest viewing or walking, compared to urban viewing or walking. Those of us who live in close proximity to a forest can spend time there taking in the sights, sounds, and smells while sitting or while walking. Our mood will likely improve, along with lowered stress, as a consequence of forest bathing[24].

Developing positive feelings with exercise, especially high degrees of pleasure and arousal, may help us *Keep Moving*. Austrian researchers investigated whether mountain walking would lead to more positive feelings than either indoor exercise or being sedentary. The researchers found that positive mood scored highest during the downhill walking portion of the mountain walking. Compared to the treadmill or sedentary conditions, mountain walking led to the largest increase in activation and elation and the greatest declines in fatigue, depression, anger, and anxiety. The greater effectiveness of the scenic mountain walking condition in promoting positive mood mirrored other studies that showed positive emotional responses to walking or otherwise being in nature. Walking in nature on a regular basis can improve our outlook on life and may encourage those of us who feel "allergic" to exercise to *Keep Moving*[25].

Another compelling study suggests we can improve our mood if we commute by bicycle instead of driving to work. Data from more than 13,000 respondents in the American Time Use Survey's well-being module were analyzed to evaluate the mood of commuters. Bicyclists had the highest degree of positive emotions compared to car riders, car drivers, and bus and train riders[26].

Better self-control

Numerous health problems arise from inadequate self-control. Australian researchers tested whether physical exercise could improve self-regulatory strength. Subjects participated in a two-month pre-program phase, during which time subjects reported perceived stress, emotional distress, and regulatory behaviors as stable. Next, the subjects entered a two-month program of regular exercise designed to increase self-regulatory strength. Compared to the pre-program phase, participants who exercised showed significant improvement in self-regulatory capacity. During the exercise phase, participants also reported significant decreases in perceived stress, emotional distress, smoking, alcohol and caffeine consumption, and increases in healthy eating, emotional control, maintenance of household chores, attendance to commitments, monitoring of spending, and improved study habits. Quite the list of positive outcomes![27].

Self-regulatory skills developed in one area, such as exercise, might spill over to others, such as eating. A study in Atlanta, Georgia, of 137 severely obese adult men and women with an average body mass index, or BMI, of 42.2, supported this idea. A BMI over 30 defines obesity. After a 26-week exercise support and nutrition program, the participants showed significant improvement in all measured factors. Changes in mood, self-regulation for *exercise*, and self-confidence with respect to *exercise* predicted significant changes in self-regulation for *eating* and self-confidence with respect to healthy *eating*. Self-confidence with respect to healthy eating and self-regulation of eating accounted for a significant portion of the variation in weight loss and waist circumference reduction. But get this: Only 12.4 percent of the observed weight loss could be attributed to increased caloric expenditure. *This is not a misprint.* Amazingly, exercise may produce weight loss mainly through improved self-regulation of eating rather than burning more calories[28].

Physical exercise reduces the craving for chocolate in people of normal weight. But does exercise provide similar benefits to overweight individuals? Researchers recruited 47 overweight people who regularly consumed sugary snacks; these subjects agreed to avoid sugary treats for three days. Half of the subjects then walked for 15 minutes. The others were passive for 15 minutes. All subjects participated in a stressful computer task and then handled several kinds of high-calorie, sweet treats. The study showed that, compared to the non-exercise control condition, a 15-minute walk reduced the urge to eat sugary snacks, the degree of emotional response to the presence of the snacks, and the emotional activation after handling sugary snacks. Thus, *Keep Moving* might help us resist the temptation to indulge in highly appealing but unhealthy snacks[29].

Improved bone health

Weight-training exercises can increase bone mineral density (BMD) in postmenopausal women. A systematic review of the literature revealed that increases in BMD required high exercise loads. For example, (1) using a weight that is 70 to 90 percent of the one-repetition maximum weight, (2) performing 8 to 12 repetitions with that weight, and (3) doing two to three sets of repetitions for (4) twice a week over one year, is an effective approach to weight training that increases BMD. Weighted exercises helped postmenopausal women increase BMD of the spine and hip, and helped women with osteopenia and osteoporosis maintain BMD. But here's the kicker: To be effective for older women, an exercise program must be incorporated as a lifelong lifestyle change[30].

Does weight-training exercise have positive effects on the bone mineral density of older men? A recent study reviewed trials examining the effect of different weight-bearing and resistance-based exercises on the BMD of hip and lumbar spine of middle-aged and older men. Effects of exercise varied greatly among studies. Resistance training alone or in combination with impact-loading activities (such as running or jumping) appeared to create the greatest benefit for bone health for older men. Walking had limited effect on BMD. Therefore, a combination of regular resistance training and impact-loading activities may help middle-aged and older men maintain bone health[31].

Maintained mobility

Most of us don't know that leg strength is the best predictor of older people being able to live on their own and to avoid being confined to a nursing home. Aging seems to reflect a progressive dysfunction of basic biological systems. Research funded under the Baltimore Longitudinal Study of Aging, one of the longest-running studies of aging in the US, shows that healthy lifestyle choices largely determine the *rate of aging*. The most important lifestyle choices appear to be *Eat Better, Keep Moving,* and *Cultivate Social Connections*. Compared to our daily choices, the genes we inherited from our parents account for a smaller proportion of our rate of aging. Poor leg strength and low leg function predict multiple bad health outcomes, including disability, greater medical care utilization, higher rate of nursing home admission, and increased mortality. Maintaining leg strength and joint capability promote mobility; maintaining a high quality of life in old age and increasing our *Quality of Lifespan* depends greatly upon maintaining that mobility[32].

Poor Outcomes Linked to a Lack of *Keep Moving*

Physical exercise is generally regarded as the single best thing we can do to eliminate or reduce the risk of conditions associated with metabolic syndrome, including abdominal obesity, hypertension, high serum triglycerides, high fasting blood glucose, and low HDL ("good") cholesterol. People who have conditions of the metabolic syndrome have greater risk for developing numerous chronic ailments, and dying prematurely, than people who lack these conditions. This section discusses 15 poor outcomes linked to a lack of *Keep Moving*.

Poor Outcomes Linked to a Lack of *Keep Moving*

- Premature death
- Cardiovascular disease
- Certain cancers
- Hypertension
- Obesity
- Type 2 diabetes
- Dementia
- Cognitive impairment and decline
- Depression
- Sarcopenia
- Disability
- Osteoporosis
- Institutionalization in a nursing home
- Upper respiratory infections
- Biological aging

Premature death

Researchers estimate that sedentary living accounts for one-third of the deaths in the U.S. due to coronary heart disease, colon cancer, and diabetes[33]. Numerous studies show that multiple health benefits associated with physical activity for younger and middle-aged persons, including reduced risk of premature death. Happily, these benefits extend to older people. Researchers in California analyzed data from 13,199 participants (average age of 87) in the Leisure World Cohort Study. The median follow-up period was 13 years. For women and men aged 70 or older at baseline, those who were active

(active outdoor plus active indoor) for more than two hours per day had a significantly lower risk of all-cause mortality than those who were active for zero hours per day. Doing something besides sitting or watching TV can help us live longer, even if we're older[34].

Cardiovascular fitness is even more important than fatness with respect to the risk of premature death. Data pooled from 10 studies showed that, compared to normal weight individuals with high cardiovascular fitness, normal weight plus poor cardiovascular fitness individuals had a 142 percent higher risk of death, regardless of BMI. Interestingly, fit yet obese individuals did not exhibit a significantly higher mortality risk compared to fit, normal weight individuals. These results suggest that poor cardiovascular fitness poses a greater risk of premature death than being obese[35].

Unquestionably, physical exercise can improve our health and promote increased longevity. But does a particular level of exercise confer the greatest benefit for longevity? Researchers in Europe performed a meta-analysis of published studies that related all causes of mortality to various types and intensities of exercise. Their analysis showed that the relative risk of death for participants with the highest activity level was 35 percent lower than for participants with the lowest activity level. The relative risks of death corresponding to 300 and 150 minutes per week of moderate and vigorous leisure-time activity (things done during free time away from work) were 26 and 14 percent lower, respectively, compared to the lowest level of activity. For vigorous exercise and sports, the comparable relative risks of death were 39 and 22 percent lower, respectively, compared to the lowest level of activity. The benefit of reduced death risk was greater for women than for men. The bottom line: More exercise is better than less, and vigorous exercise is better than moderate exercise or vigorous leisure-time activity to reduce the risk of premature death[36].

A meta-analysis is a statistical procedure that includes several to many separate but similar experiments. The larger resulting sample sizes increases the likelihood that a meta-analysis can detect real outcomes, such as the link between some type of physical activity and the risk of premature death.

Cardiovascular disease

Cardiovascular disease kills more people in the U.S. than any other cause. Research shows that physical exercise increases cardiovascular fitness and can reduce the risk of heart disease and stroke by more than 50 percent[37]. Many people don't realize that cardiovascular disease occurs mainly in the arteries of un-muscled parts of the body where the lymphatic system transports lipids (fat molecules), including LDL ("bad") cholesterol and oxidized LDL cholesterol. The latter is implicated in arterial plaque formation. Unlike blood, lymph has no pump to move it around the body. Rather, bodily movements power the lymphatic system. Sedentary people may have compromised lymphatic transport. This can lead to oxidized LDL cholesterol remaining in the arteries rather than being transported to the liver for reprocessing[38].

Researchers with the Honolulu Heart Program investigated whether walking reduced the risk of coronary heart disease. They followed 2,678 men aged 71–93 at baseline for two to four years. The risk of coronary heart disease declined by 15 percent for each 0.5-mile increase in distance walked per day[39]. Men who walked 0.9 miles per day had a 2.6 times greater risk of coronary heart disease compared to men who walked 2.1–8.0 miles per day.

Stroke is a particularly debilitating type of cardiovascular disease and the third leading cause of death in the U.S. How important is cardiovascular fitness in predicting fatal and non-fatal strokes in men and women? Researchers addressed this question using data from a longitudinal research study at the Cooper Clinic in Dallas, Texas. The patients (46,505 men and 15,282 women) came to the clinic over 31 years for preventive health exams and counseling regarding lifestyle factors associated with an increased risk of chronic diseases. The findings revealed that men in the highest quartile of cardiovascular fitness had a 50–52 percent lower risk for fatal stroke and a 38–49 percent lower risk for non-fatal stroke, respectively, compared to men in the lowest quartile of fitness. For women, the comparable reductions in risk were 56–67 percent for fatal stroke and 44–49 percent for non-fatal stroke. The incidence of stroke dropped substantially for men or women who achieved more than 7.5 metabolic equivalents, or METs, on their treadmill test. A level of 7–8 METs reflects a low to moderate level of cardiovascular fitness. Thus, if we achieve a moderate level of cardiovascular fitness, we may substantially reduce our risk of fatal or non-fatal stroke[40].

METs (metabolic equivalents) measure the ratio of the amount of energy required to perform a task to the amount of energy expended while resting. One MET is defined roughly as the energy of sitting quietly. A higher MET means a higher rate of energy expenditure.

Physical activity is the most widely recommended means of reducing the risk of coronary heart disease. But few studies have evaluated lifetime activity patterns and their association with this disease. Researchers reanalyzed data from a previously published study investigating lifetime patterns. Their findings were encouraging. Compared to persons who were rarely or slightly active during all three age periods (20–39, 40–49, and 50 years and older), those who were rarely or a little active at ages 20–39 but became very active thereafter had only a 10 percent risk of coronary heart disease. Thus, intense physical activity after age 40 appeared to dramatically reduce the risk of coronary heart disease, even for people who were previously sedentary[41]. Those of us who are 50-year-old couch potatoes can rejuvenate our cardiovascular system with vigorous exercise. It's never too late to enjoy the benefits of *Keep Moving*.

Certain cancers

In 2007, Polish physical education researcher Joanna Kruk reviewed evidence supporting the strongest positive influence of physical activity upon preventing colon cancer, breast cancer, and cardiovascular disease. Since then, additional evidence has accumulated, documenting the beneficial effects of *Keep Moving* for cancer and other chronic conditions[42]. An updated report in 2012 by the World Cancer Research Fund/American Institute for Cancer Research Continuous Project found convincing evidence that physical activity protects against colon cancer[43].

The relationships between leisure-time physical activity and cancer are not as well established as they are for cardiovascular health and all-cause mortality. However, a new study using pooled data from a dozen observational studies from the U.S. and Europe examined this relationship. With the resulting large sample size (1.44 million adults), enough incidences of cancer occurred to reveal links between leisure-time physical activity and risk reduction in different types of cancer. Of the 26 types of cancer studied, positive and statistically significant associations were found for 15 cancers, no significant association was found for nine cancers, and negative and statistically insignificant associations were found for two cancers. The five cancers with the highest observed reduction in risk for subjects in the higher activity/most active group included esophageal adenocarcinoma (42 percent), gallbladder (38 percent), liver (27 percent), lung (26 percent), and kidney (23 percent). Overall, the higher activity/most active subjects had a 7-percentage-point lower risk in absolute terms on any type of cancer compared to lower activity/less active subjects. Thus, there appears to be little doubt that leisure-time physical exercise predicts modestly lower incidence of cancer[44].

Hypertension

Hypertension, commonly known as high blood pressure, is a well-established risk factor for cardiovascular disease. Blood pressure typically rises with age. The American College of Sports Medicine recommends 30 minutes of moderate-intensity exercise at least five times per week. But is that enough to lower blood pressure in older people? Researchers at the University of Tennessee recruited 24 postmenopausal women with borderline or stage 1 hypertension (systolic blood pressure of 130–139 mm Hg, diastolic blood pressure of 80–89 mm Hg) for an exercise experiment. Over 24 weeks, women in the exercise group walked 1.8 miles per day above their regular amount of walking; the women in the control group did not change their activity. After 12 weeks, the women in the exercise group reduced their systolic blood pressure by an average of 6 mm Hg; after another 12 weeks, these women reduced their average blood pressure by another 5 mm Hg. Women in the control group did not show any change in blood pressure at either 12 or 24 weeks. Reducing systolic blood pressure by 11 mm Hg is clinically significant. Six of the women in the exercise group normalized their blood pressure, versus none in the control group. Thus, daily walking that meets the American College of Sports Medicine recommendation effectively lowered blood pressure in postmenopausal, borderline hypertensive women[45]. Trading 30 minutes of watching TV or surfing the web for 30 minutes of walking five days a week could dramatically reduce our risk of hypertension and cardiovascular disease.

Researchers in Australia addressed the extent to which physical activity affected the risk of overweight or obese individuals developing hypertension. Study participants included 9,217 middle-aged women born between 1946 and 1951 with no history of hypertension; participants were followed for 14 years. Women with no physical activity had a 59 percent higher risk of hypertension than women with a high level of physical activity[46].

Obesity

The prevalence of obesity in the U.S. increased dramatically over the past few decades. Between 1960 and 2002, Americans aged 20–29 expanded from 128 to 157 pounds, an average increase of 29 pounds. Those aged 40–49 grew from 142 to 169 pounds, an average gain of 27 pounds. Weight gains were greatest among the heaviest people[47].

Many health experts regard obesity as the leading public health challenge facing the U.S. However, obesity is a problem not only in the U.S. but also in other countries, such as Brazil. The Household Budget Survey 2008–2009 showed that 50.1 percent of adult men in Brazil were overweight and 12.4 percent were obese. Researchers used pedometers to study the walking habits of 299 men between ages 40 and 59 who worked in various office jobs at the Federal University of Vicosa, Brazil. The results showed a relationship between the number of steps walked and cardiovascular risk factors. Subjects who walked more than 10,000 steps per day had a lower body mass index, less abdominal fat, and lower insulin and triglyceride levels. The take-home message: Apparently healthy middle-aged Brazilian men who walked more than 10,000 steps per day exhibited better cardiovascular health and less evidence of metabolic syndrome than men who walked fewer than 10,000 steps daily[48].

Type 2 diabetes

The worldwide incidence of type 2 diabetes increased greatly in recent years[49]. Diabetics run a greater risk of serious complications, including amputations, blindness, and kidney failure, than non-diabetics.

Physical exercise provides diabetics with well-known health benefits. Researchers at Louisiana State University and elsewhere designed a study to test whether combining resistance training with aerobic training would reduce risk factors for type 2 diabetes more than doing either type of physical activity alone. The researchers found that patients who engaged in both resistance and aerobic training reduced their levels of HbA1c (glycated hemoglobin)—a measure of average blood sugar levels over two to three months—more than patients in the aerobic exercise or resistance training or non-exercise control groups. In addition, people in all the exercise groups (resistance training, aerobic training, or combined resistance training and aerobic training) displayed reduced waist circumference. People in the resistance training and combined training groups lost more weight, on average, than people in the control group. The combination of resistance and aerobic training provided more protection against type 2 diabetes than either resistance or aerobic training or no exercise[50].

Studies suggest that physical inactivity is an independent risk factor for excess abdominal fat. Belly fat is different from other fat in that it activates chronic inflammation, which promotes insulin resistance—the decreased ability of the body to use insulin to move glucose out of the blood and into cells—among other ills. The protective effect of exercise may partly arise from its anti-inflammatory effect. Muscles activated by physical exercise produce and release small proteins called myokines, which may exert hormone-like effects that help metabolize abdominal fat[51].

Insulin resistance, or reduced insulin sensitivity, which is linked to the onset of type 2 diabetes, is commonly regarded as an inevitable consequence of aging. Endurance training increases insulin sensitivity in short-term studies. But does endurance training promote insulin sensitivity, offsetting the effects of aging, over the long term? Researchers at the Mayo Clinic recruited 22 healthy younger subjects (ages 18–30) and 20 healthy older subjects (ages 59–76) and divided them into four groups: young endurance-trained, young sedentary, older endurance-trained, and older sedentary. The researchers found that both the young and older endurance-trained subjects had greater insulin sensitivity than the sedentary subjects, regardless of age. Insulin sensitivity did not decline with age for the endurance-trained/physically active subjects. The great news from this study: A decline in insulin sensitivity with age is actually caused by physical inactivity and fat deposition rather than age itself[52]. We can maintain insulin sensitivity and greatly reduce our risk of type 2 diabetes if we *Keep Moving*.

Dementia

Half of today's 70-year-old baby boomers who live to their expected age of 85 are projected to develop Alzheimer's disease (AD). Physical exercise is currently regarded as the best thing we can do to reduce our risk of AD. According to University of Washington researcher John Medina, author of *Brain Rules*, aerobic physical exercise can reduce the risk of getting AD by more than 60 percent.

Two researchers reviewed evidence regarding seven potentially modifiable risk factors for AD and determined that up to half of all AD cases may be attributable to those factors. In the U.S., physical inactivity accounted for the greatest proportion of AD cases[53]. If we embrace the healthy choice of *Keep Moving*, we'll likely lower our risk of AD.

Both physical activity and diet independently predict risk of AD. While their joint effects are poorly understood, researchers have observed that physical activity appears to confer more protection against AD than adopting a Mediterranean diet. Therefore, even a little physical activity might help forestall or eliminate AD[54].

In 2015, an estimated 5.3 million Americans had AD. Total payments for health care, long-term care, and hospice care for patients age 65 and older with dementia totaled roughly $226 billion[55]. By 2050, the number of Americans with AD is projected to increase by 10 million. Dementia exacts a major financial burden upon America, while the emotional cost of caring for a loved one with dementia can be even greater[56].

Cognitive impairment and decline

Cognitive impairment is a mild but measurable form of dementia that doesn't unduly limit activities of daily living. However, cognitive impairment, common in older people, is a risk factor for more severe forms of dementia. Lack of physical activity has been suggested as a possible risk factor that we can control. Possible mechanisms by which physical activity might improve cognition include increased cerebral blood flow, reduced risk of cardiovascular disease, and increased nerve cell growth. Researchers analyzed data collected from 5,925 community-dwelling women (average age of 70) enrolled in the Study of Osteoporotic Fractures. At the end of the follow-up period (six to eight years), women who had walked the fewest number of blocks per week and expended the least amount of energy per week were much more likely to exhibit cognitive decline. If we *Keep Moving*, we may reduce our risk of cognitive decline later in life[57].

Stave Off Depression and Cardiovascular Disease with Exercise

Major depression is an established risk factor for cardiovascular disease. Possible mechanisms of a cause-and-effect relationship include a reduced adoption of healthy lifestyle choices by depressed persons and direct physiological effects. The established benefits of exercise for reducing the risk of depression and, presumably, the risk of cardiovascular disease, should motivate the medical community to develop inexpensive hospital or community exercise programs that provide home- or group-based social support and coaching. Such programs could be designed to increase patient autonomy, self-efficacy, and self-monitoring, all of which promote healthy behaviors. The upside for such programs is potentially enormous, given that both depression and cardiovascular disease cost Americans hundreds of billions of dollars annually, while also causing great pain and suffering[59].

Depression

A group of researchers devised a controlled experiment to determine whether aerobic exercise is an effective treatment for mild to moderate depression. Subjects included 80 sedentary persons (ages 20–45 years) with mild to moderate depression. These subjects were randomly assigned to one of four groups: 1) high energy expenditure and exercising three days per week, 2) high energy expenditure and exercising five days per week, 3) low energy expenditure and exercising three days per week, and 4) low energy expenditure and exercising five days per week. A stretching group served as a control. The high-energy level corresponded to public health recommendations for physical activity. After 12 weeks, subjects in the high-energy expenditure groups had significantly lower depression than subjects in the low-energy expenditure or control groups, regardless of exercise frequency. Improvement in depressive symptoms for people in the high-energy groups was comparable to symptoms observed in other studies where subjects took medication. Furthermore, the rate of adherence or compliance for the persons in the high-energy groups was comparable to that in medication trials[58].

Depression is a major health issue for older people, affecting approximately 7-10 percent of community dwellers and 18 percent of nursing home residents. Major depressive disorder also predicts higher mortality risk. Motivated by previous studies, researchers conducted a randomized, controlled trial to compare the effectiveness of physical exercise versus medication in treating major depressive disorder. Researchers assigned 100 patients age 50 or older to one of three treatment groups: medication (sertraline, which is sold under the trade name of Zoloft, among others), physical exercise, or medication and exercise. After 16 weeks, all three treatments reduced the severity of depressive symptoms. Importantly, 60 percent of the exercise group, 66 percent of the combined group, and 69 percent of the medication patients no longer met the criteria for major depressive disorder. While patients who received medication improved faster than those who engaged in physical exercise, differences were not statistically significant at 16 weeks[60].

Structured aerobic exercise in a supervised setting may be as effective as medication in treating major depressive disorder—but without the side effects of medication.

Sarcopenia

Sarcopenia (bodily wasting) is a syndrome characterized by progressive, generalized loss of skeletal muscle and strength. Sarcopenia predicts a higher risk of physical disability, reduced *Quality of Lifespan*, higher health care costs, and premature death. Who wants any of those? The origins of sarcopenia are not completely clear, but physical inactivity and poor diet appear to be key factors. Resistance exercise is especially effective in preventing, slowing, and reversing sarcopenia[61]. Thus, we can likely reduce our risk of sarcopenia by adopting two healthy choices: *Keep Moving* and *Eat Better*.

Human aging is associated with progressive muscle weakness and functional impairment. Mitochondrial dysfunction—the inability of mitochondria to break down nutrients in our cells to release energy— appears to contribute to muscle deterioration and sarcopenia. If that's the case, mitochondrial gene expression would likely differ between young and old adults. Researchers collected leg muscle tissue samples recruited 26 apparently healthy, relatively inactive younger adults and 25 apparently healthy, relatively active older adults who participated in a related study. Fourteen of the older subjects (but none of the younger subjects) participated in a 26-week, whole-body, progressive resistance-training program. Prior to exercise training, the older adults had an average of 59 percent lower strength in their quadriceps, a group of muscles on the front of the thigh, than the younger adults. But after resistance training, that gap narrowed to 39 percent.

During the study, researchers identified 596 genes from leg muscle that expressed differentially with age. Prior to the 26 weeks of resistance training, the gene expression profile was associated with aged mitochondrial function. After the training, the gene expression profile of older, weight-trained subjects shifted mostly to that of younger ages. Healthy older adults typically show signs of muscle weakness and mitochondrial impairment. But both can be partially reversed at the leg-strength and gene-expression levels with resistance training over a period of six months. Older adults can reduce their risk of sarcopenia through strength training[62].

Disability

Disability in old age can shorten *Quality of Lifespan*. Decreased muscle strength predicts disability and functional limitations. Would long-time running (average of 12.4 years) protect older people from disability? James Fries and his colleagues at Stanford University studied members of a running club in California. The Runners Study began in 1984 and followed 523 senior men and women runners (average age of 58) with a control group of age-matched non-runners. Over an eight-year period, the disability of the women and men non-runners in the control group diverged significantly from that of the women and men runners. Disability of the runners increased only between ages 75 and 79. The mortality for runners was also significantly lower than for the non-runners, resulting in an estimated two years of extra longevity for the former group. Exercise appears to be a key aspect of prolonging a disability-free life and increasing our *Quality of Lifespan*[63].

Fries and colleagues reexamined the surviving members of the Runners Study 18 years later. Over 25 years, through an average age of 80, the differences in disability between the runners and non-runners steadily increased. Relative to the non-runners, the runners postponed mild disability for four years and moderate disability for 16 years. Runners also enjoyed longer lives than non-runners. At year 25 of the study, runners experienced a 40 percent lower mortality risk than non-runners[64].

Physical activity is widely regarded as a key aspect of lifelong health and well-being. But does physical activity help prevent disability arising from mobility limitations in older adults? The Lifestyle Interventions and Independence for Elders (LIFE) study addressed this question. Investigators randomized a sample of 1,635 sedentary men and women to either a physical activity group or a health education program group. Follow-up continued for an average of 2.6 years. The physical activity intervention included walking (with a goal of 150 minutes per week), strength training, and flexibility training. Physical activity group participants attended two fitness-center-based sessions per week and engaged in home-based activity three to four times per week. Persons in the health education group attended weekly health education workshops for 26 weeks, then monthly sessions thereafter. Compared to those in the health education group, those in the physical activity group had an 18 percent lower risk of major mobility disability and a 28 percent lower risk of persistent mobility disability. Given the severe impact of mobility disability on well-being, a physical activity program for older adults could reduce the risk of disability and increase *Quality of Lifespan*[65].

Osteoporosis

Osteoporosis affects more than 14 million Americans, especially postmenopausal women. This condition involves the loss of bone mass and a reduction in bone quality and strength. Physical activity and diet (primarily vitamin D and calcium intake) appear to be the key factors that prevent osteoporosis. It's important to remember that bone isn't static; rather, like all bodily tissues, bone remodeling occurs constantly. As such, bone adapts positively to stresses arising from physical activity.

A recent review evaluated different types of physical activity with respect to their ability to prevent osteoporosis in postmenopausal women. The two most effective ways to stimulate bone metabolism and increase bone strength were impact exercises and resistance exercises. Impact activities, such as running, jumping rope, and stair climbing, appeared to be most beneficial. Resistance exercises, such as weight lifting, exercise bands, and plyometrics (jump training), seemed to be less beneficial. Dynamic, short-duration, high-intensity exercises provided the greatest benefit. Strengthening back extensor muscles appeared to be especially valuable in supporting the spine. Walking on level surfaces at a moderate pace, although valuable for improving general health, was less effective for preventing osteoporosis. Faster walking on rocky surfaces would seem to provide greater benefit than slower walking on level surfaces. High-impact aquatic exercise, yoga, and tai chi can improve body balance and reduce falls, thus mitigating some of the negative effects of osteoporosis[66].

Institutionalization in a nursing home

Seniors fear losing their independence and being confined to a nursing home more than they fear dying, according to a study, "Aging in Place in America." Hip fractures are a major cause of nursing home admission. Studies indicate that physical exercise reduces the risk of falls and the risk of hip fractures resulting from falls.

Which type, intensity, and duration of exercise reduces the risk of a hip fracture? Researchers at Harvard used data from 121,700 women nurses in the Nurses' Health Study to investigate this question.

Compared to postmenopausal women in the lowest category of activity (< 3 MET-hours per week), those in the highest category of activity (> 24 MET-hours per week) had only a 38 to 45 percent of the risk of hip fracture, depending on which statistical model was used. Women who reported low activity in 1980 (less than one hour per week) but who increased activity to at least four hours per week by 1986 had a 57 percent lower risk of hip fracture than women who remained in the low-activity category. Thus, even during later adult years, increasing physical activity predicted a reduced risk of hip fracture in women. However, the activity (brisk walking 30–60 minutes per day) needed to be sustained to maintain the benefit[67].

Increasing physical activity also reduces the risk of hip fractures in men. A subset of the Finnish Twin Cohort looked at same-sex twins born in Finland before 1938 with both co-twins alive in 1967. When the study began in 1975, it included 3,262 men age 44 or older who were free of debilitating medical and/or physical conditions. The follow-up period lasted 21 years, and examined hip fractures resulting from minimal trauma, such as falling from a standing height. The age-adjusted risk of hip fracture in men participating in vigorous physical activity was 62 percent lower than that of men who did not engage in strenuous physical activity. Moderate to high levels of physical activity can reduce the risk of hip fracture for men[68].

Physical weakness is commonly regarded as an inevitable part of old age, often resulting in elderly people being confined to a nursing home due to their inability to physically handle the activities of daily life. But research suggests that physical weakness can be reversed. Volunteers living in a long-term care facility participated in a study to determine if lower-body-resistance exercise and nutrient supplementation could improve their strength and functional capabilities. The 94 subjects who completed the 12-week study had an average age of 87. Nearly all required a cane, walker, or wheelchair to move about at baseline. The findings were impressive. Subjects who exercised increased their lower body muscle strength by 113 percent on average, while those who did not exercise increased their muscle strength by 3 percent. Gait velocity, stair climbing ability, and overall physical activity increased dramatically in the subjects who exercised, compared to those who did not. The cross-sectional area of the thigh muscles increased by 2.7 percent and decreased by 1.8 percent in the exercise and non-exercise groups, respectively. The modest increase in the size of the thigh muscle, compared with the much larger increase in lower-body strength, suggested that improved utilization of existing but underused muscles created most of the observed increase in strength. Older people can use progressive strength training to delay or eliminate the onset of frailty[69], thereby reducing the risk of nursing home admissions.

While physical activity benefits older people, can it help people with existing mobility impairment reduce the risk of becoming dependent or dying prematurely? Researchers studied 1,109 independently-living residents in Jyvaskyla, Finland, between the ages of 65 and 84 at baseline, and again eight years later. Physical inactivity and impaired mobility after baseline predicted subsequent dependence and earlier death in both men and women. Men who were mobility-impaired at baseline had about four times the risk of losing their independence, compared to men who were not mobility-impaired at baseline. But being physically active predicted a lower risk of becoming dependent. Therefore, older people with mobility impairment can reduce their risk of further mobility impairment by becoming physically active[70].

Upper respiratory infections

An upper respiratory tract infection (URTI) is not as earthshaking as cancer, though it exacts a substantial toll on the U.S. economy, estimated at $40 billion annually. Plus having a runny nose and sneezing on your friends isn't much fun for you or them. Studies prior to 2010 lacked validated measures to assess URTI incidence and severity. In a more recent study that followed a validated protocol, roughly 1,000 male and female subjects completed a 12-week study designed to test whether physical fitness and aerobic activity were associated with the frequency of upper respiratory infections. Participants in the highest one-third level of physical fitness exhibited URTI symptoms for 46 percent fewer days than participants in the lowest one-third level of physical fitness. Similarly, participants in the highest one-third of aerobic activity exhibited URTI symptoms for 43 percent fewer days than participants in the lowest one-third of aerobic activity [71]. This study confirms results of other studies: Regular exercise can reduce the risk of colds and flu.

Biological aging

Confusion exists regarding the inevitability of biological aging for older adults. Understanding the difference between primary aging and secondary aging provides clarity. Primary aging refers to progressive, inevitable bodily deterioration during adulthood. Secondary aging refers to deterioration that arises from diseases and lifestyle choices. Much of secondary aging can be reduced or postponed with better lifestyle choices. Exercise can thwart secondary aging by maintaining mitochondrial function and muscle mass. Both physical activity (related to daily activities) and exercise (planned activities to improve body condition) can increase longevity, and, more importantly, increase *Quality of Lifespan*. Insufficient bodily movement leads to a host of undesirable bodily changes, including muscle atrophy, loss of muscle mass, fat accumulation, reduced insulin sensitivity, impaired glucose tolerance, and type 2 diabetes. Loss of muscle mass is also associated with functional decline and increases in disability and dependence.

In one study, a group of 67-year-old women who walked briskly for one hour showed increased insulin sensitivity the very next day. (Talk about quick positive results!) Endurance exercise performed three to five times weekly improved insulin sensitivity and reduced body fat in just a few weeks[72].

Two-thirds of Americans aged 60–74 have diabetes (mostly type 2), abnormal blood glucose levels, and impaired glucose tolerance. The prevalence of these three conditions rises to three-quarters for Americans at least 75 years-old. These data suggest a looming public health disaster, given that by 2060 Americans over age 65 will account for roughly 24 percent of the US population[73]. On the other hand, the proverbial "fountain of youth" may be just down the street at our neighborhood gym[74]. *Keep Moving is huge, especially for older people!*

How we age is also linked to the length of telomeres, the protective caps that cover the ends of chromosomes and promote their stability. As our cells divide, telomeres shorten, eventually resulting in cellular death. Thus, minimizing the rate of telomere shortening may reduce the rate of cellular aging. Chronic psychological stress is linked to shorter telomeres. Researchers at the University of California, San Francisco, wanted to know whether physical activity could maintain telomere length by reducing chronic stress. They recruited 63, apparently healthy, postmenopausal women (ages 54–82) with varying levels of self-reported stress. Each subject donated a blood sample (telomere length was measured for white blood cells), filled out a 10-item psychological stress questionnaire, and reported the number of minutes of vigorous physical exercise for three consecutive days. The probability of short telomere length increased with perceived stress, but *only for the sedentary subjects*. Physical exercise appeared to mitigate the adverse effect of perceived psychological stress on telomere length. Thus, *Keep Moving* may indirectly help slow biological aging[75].

Bed rest leads to reduced physiological function, much like aging. In 1966, five 20-year-old men participated in a study of their ability to recover from three weeks of bed rest by means of eight weeks of intensive endurance training. The same five men were re-evaluated 30 and 40 years later. As expected, their average ability to process oxygen (VO_2 max) declined over time. The average decline in VO_2 max over 40 years was comparable to that observed after three weeks of bed rest. Forty years after three weeks of bed rest, the oxygen processing abilities of the men varied greatly. In fact, one of the men had the same VO_2 max at age 60 as he had at age 20! Thus, oxygen processing ability usually but not always declines with chronological aging[76].

Practical Ways to *Keep Moving*

- **Trade 30 minutes of TV or computer time for 30 minutes of movement.** Shifting a half hour of your daily time ledger from the sedentary to the physical activity side provides double benefits—less time sitting and more time moving. Metabolic risk factors increase as the length of daily TV watching increases. These risk factors include waist circumference, systolic blood pressure, and blood glucose in both men and women[77]. You'll likely be healthier if you curb your sedentary periods, including TV viewing.

- **Set your watch or computer to beep every hour or half hour while working at your desk or while typing on your computer.** After each beep, spend two minutes doing something besides sitting to reduce your risk of type 2 diabetes and cardiovascular disease. You could go to the bathroom, walk outside to check the weather, or walk up a set of stairs and come back down. You'll also feel rejuvenated[78].

- **Develop the healthy habit of taking a brisk 22-minute walk every day after dinner**. Walks beginning 30 minutes after a meal help keep blood sugar under control, potentially reducing the risk of type 2 diabetes. My wife and I take a 22-minute walk nearly every day—rain or shine—after dinner. We enjoy the fresh air and often chat with neighbors. Plus it guarantees that we'll get the recommended 150 minutes of moderate-intensity exercise each week.

- **Tend a garden.** The physical activity of tending a garden counts toward your daily exercise needs. In addition, you can enjoy the taste and the nutritional benefits of garden-fresh produce during the warmer months. All winter long, my wife and I eat pesto that she lovingly made from our home-grown basil. Yum! Plus we give it away as presents.

- **Walk a dog.** If you have a dog, do the dog and yourself a favor and walk your pooch at least twice a day. Two brisk 22-minute walks can get you the minimum amount of recommended daily exercise. Plus, you'll *Cultivate Social Connections*, another key healthy choice.

- **Run errands on foot or on your bicycle**. When possible, walk or bike to the bank, library, gym, office supply store, and grocery store. Several years ago, I attended a class sponsored by a local cycling group. All attendees received a recycled, heavy-duty kitty litter box (plus hardware) that we attached to our bikes—this in lieu of a smaller standard bike basket. Since then, I've greatly increased the number of errands I run on my bike rather than in my car. These days, I prefer running errands by bike.

- **Join a fitness club.** Many people resist going to the gym—they might feel insecure or uneasy, or perhaps they don't want to pay for a membership. Many of the regulars at the YMCA where I exercise are not models of physical fitness. They look like normal people. But they show up and do the work. You can too. Fitness clubs have staff members who can show you how to use the equipment safely. Personal trainers can create a customized exercise routine at low cost. If you're enrolled in a Medicare supplemental plan, you may be eligible for a free Silver Sneakers gym membership.

- **Incorporate movement into your vacations.** Rather than lying on the beach all the time and eating too much, find opportunities to *Keep Moving*. Do your homework and look for places to ride a bicycle, hike, swim, or workout at a local gym. My YMCA membership gets me into YMCAs all across America.

- **Incorporate movement into your business travel.** Rather than sitting in meetings all day and then eating too much rich food, find opportunities to *Keep Moving*. Maybe the best you can do is to use the exercise facility at the hotel. Call ahead to make sure the hotel has an exercise room that's suitable. Perhaps you can find a place to take a walk with some of your work colleagues. Or find a pool and swim laps.

- **Try interval training.** Martin Gibala and his colleagues at McMaster University in Ontario, Canada, conducted numerous studies of the health effects of interval training. This approach to *Keep Moving* features short, alternating periods of intense exercise and recovery within a single training session. Interval training provides a time-efficient way to improve cardiovascular fitness. A new study by Gibala and colleagues tested whether extra-short bouts of stair climbing would lead to improved cardiovascular performance. Indeed, sedentary young adults who performed three sets of fast-as-possible stair climbing (each lasting 20 seconds with each climb separated by one to four hours) for three days per week for six weeks increased their peak oxygen uptake compared to a non-training control group. If you think you don't have enough time to improve your cardiovascular health, think of this study then start climbing the stairs at work[79].

Three Points to Remember

1. *Keep Moving may be the most important thing you can do* to create and maintain a healthy body.

2. Ideally, *Keep Moving* includes aerobic, strength building, flexibility, and balance activities.

3. Adding even a little movement into your daily life will nurture your body; more is better.

Chapter 2

Eat Better

Let us think of life as a process of choices, one after another.
—Abraham Maslow

Of the nine healthy lifestyle choices, *Eat Better* might be the least settled from scientific research and clinical standpoints. People respond differently to certain foods, possibly accounting in part for conflicting opinions regarding a healthy diet. While there is no magic bullet, and no single combination of foods can best achieve and maintain wellness for everyone, recent research generally supports the following recommendations: (1) minimize sugary drinks, (2) eat less white flour in its many guises, (3) eat more vegetables (especially the non-starchy kinds) and fruits, and (4) eat more fiber. Within these broad guidelines, we have wide latitude to choose foods that we enjoy eating, find satisfying, and which we believe support our health and well-being. You'll find more detailed information about specific foods later in this chapter.

Notwithstanding the uncertainty of exactly which foods comprise *Eat Better* for a particular person, researchers agree that what we eat strongly affects our health and how we feel. This chapter makes the case that those of us who *Eat Better* will enjoy numerous benefits, while those who follow the standard American diet will likely experience poor health outcomes. While it's tempting to buy into the hype of enticing food labels and trends *du jour*, the key to *Eat Better* involves making small changes to our daily eating choices that we will continue to make over time.

Evolutionary Perspectives on the Human Diet

Approximately 10,000 years ago, the development of agriculture ushered in a new food age for humanity. More recently, the Industrial Revolution caused drastic changes in what people ate. Today, most foods typically consumed in Western countries bear little resemblance to those of our ancient ancestors. *Paleo Diet* author Loren Cordain and colleagues contend that modern humans haven't had sufficient time to adapt to such dramatic dietary changes[1]. This disparity—between our evolutionary experience of eating mostly wild plants and meat and our modern "standard American diet" of processed foods—appears to underpin chronic diseases that plague Western countries.

The evolutionary "template" of humans predicts that optimal gene expression and, ultimately, vibrant health over our lifespan won't occur by adopting any single dietary or lifestyle change. Instead, we can adopt a combination of measures that mimic the lives of our ancient ancestors, including regular physical exercise, relaxation, sensible sun exposure, adequate sleep, avoidance of tobacco, reduced exposure to pollutants, reduced frying and grilling of foods[2].

Approaches to *Eat Better*

Americans spend billions of dollars on diet plans to lose weight. "Dieting," that is, restricting food intake to lose weight, typically leads to short-term weight loss. Unfortunately, few dieters keep the weight off and become healthier over the long term. In fact, after several years, many dieters end up weighing more than they weighed prior to starting their first diet. Additionally, weight cycling, which arises from repeated bouts of dieting, may lead to increased risk of heart attack, stroke, and type 2 diabetes[3]. Some health researchers now suggest that doctors who prescribe diets violate their Hippocratic oath, "First do no harm," given that diets are typically ineffective and counterproductive over the long term[4].

Given the unsatisfactory track record of dieting, we need a better approach to selecting and eating foods that nourish the body. Three alternative approaches merit our attention. The first approach is described in the groundbreaking book *Intuitive Eating: A Revolutionary Program that Works* by Evelyn Tribole and Elyse Resch[5]. The authors developed the intuitive eating approach based on decades of experience as nutritionists and nutrition therapists. Intuitive eating rests on the premises that we can enjoy what we eat and simultaneously monitor the physical and emotional effects of what we eat. The result is eating in a way that's both satisfying and healthful. Eating is not just a means of refueling our body; it encompasses a host of emotional experiences, especially feelings about body image. In addition, many of us eat to cope with stress, but potentially at a significant cost to our health.

The second alternative, the trust model, was developed by dietician and social worker Ellyn Satter in her book *Your Child's Weight: Helping without Harming*[6]. Analogous to intuitive eating, the trust model is based on the premise that children can self-regulate food intake by recognizing hunger, appetite and fullness cues. The trust model assigns parents the responsibility to plan and serve meals which include protein, carbohydrates, fruits, vegetables, calcium, and fat. The child's responsibility is to decide what and how much to eat from the variety of foods provided. Similar to intuitive eating, the trust model de-emphasizes: (1) counting calories, (2) eliminating certain foods, and (3) relying on low-fat or low-calorie foods[7].

The third approach is mindfulness training, which focuses on psychological aspects of habit formation to help change our relationship with food. Modern American environments often feature large amounts of "hyperpalatable" foods, so-called because they're irresistible. Repeated consumption of such foods can rewire the brain, creating a powerful reward structure. Modern eating occurs largely in response to external cues (such as the presence of hyperpalatable food or stressors) rather than internal cues (hunger, satiety, and satisfaction). Recent research shows that mindfulness training can help smokers stop smoking and reduce craving-induced eating. Successful eating-related mindfulness training follows these three steps: (1) becoming aware of habitual eating patterns and factors that trigger them, (2) understanding clearly the true immediate "rewards" of our habits (which may not be desirable), and (3) making unforced, personal choices about food. Accepting our current eating situation with a sense of curiosity, self-compassion, and a lack of judgment underlies mindfulness training[8].

Food cravings strongly predict uncontrolled eating, which may lead to overweight and obesity. Researchers tested a mobile phone app that delivered a self-paced 28-day mindfulness-based program targeting food cravings in a group of 104 overweight and obese women. The program sought to decouple the experiences of craving and eating via: (1) focusing awareness on habitual behavior, to identify triggers that support the habit of uncontrolled eating; (2) acknowledging the outcome(s) of this habit; and (3) learning to acknowledge and exist with cravings until they subside. In essence, this program sought to help participants develop a nonjudgmental awareness of their eating experiences. Those who completed the program experienced significant reduction of food cravings and craving-related eating. Changing our relationship with food through mindfulness may help us *Eat Better* and enjoy better health and well-being[9].

A recent systematic review evaluated 18 published articles of non-diet interventions for better eating. None of the studies found worsening markers of ill health (blood pressure, blood glucose, cholesterol). Non-diet, weight neutral interventions predicted significant improvements in disordered eating, self-esteem, and depression, and show promise in improving physical and mental health[10].

Benefits of *Eat Better*

Eat Better is a powerful lifestyle choice that figures prominently into our health and wellness. The following list includes nine benefits linked to *Eat Better.*

Benefits Linked to Eat Better

- Reduced risk of cardiovascular disease
- Better blood sugar control
- Reduced risk of diabetes
- Reduced risk of Alzheimer's disease
- Reduced risk of some cancers
- Improved cognitive function and brain health
- Reduced risk of cognitive decline
- Improved microbiome health
- Reduced body fat

Reduced risk of cardiovascular disease

Observational studies and randomized trials suggest that a Mediterranean-style diet reduces the risk of cardiovascular disease and/or type 2 diabetes. While there is no universally agreed-upon definition of Mediterranean diet, most researchers list abundant vegetables, fruits, nuts, fish, legumes, and olive oil as typical constituents. Consider the PREDIMED study in Spain. A total of 7,447 men and women (ages 55 to 85) with major cardiovascular disease risk factors were randomized into one of three groups: (1) Mediterranean diet plus extra-virgin olive oil, (2) Mediterranean diet plus nuts, or (3) a control diet, with reduced fat intake. The average follow-up period was 4.8 years when the trial was stopped because the results were so compelling. Subjects in the Mediterranean diet plus olive oil and the Mediterranean diet plus nuts groups had a 29 percent lower risk of cardiovascular events (heart attack, stroke, or death) than subjects in the control diet group. The researchers attributed the health benefits of the Mediterranean diet mainly to the extra-virgin olive oil and nut consumption. Numerous studies suggest that olive oil may reduce the risk of cardiovascular disease and other chronic diseases. Of note: The baseline diet of most participants (including those in the control group) was similar to a Mediterranean diet. Thus, the health advantage of a Mediterranean-type diet might be even greater for those who eat the standard American diet[11].

Americans would benefit from a Mediterranean diet, according to 12 years of data from 25,994 participants in the Women's Health Study. Compared to participants with low adherence to a Mediterranean diet, those with medium or high adherences had 23 and 28 percent lower risks of new cardiovascular disease, respectively. The four largest mediators of cardiovascular disease risk reduction in relation to Mediterranean diet adherence included: (1) markers of bio-inflammation, (2) glucose metabolism and insulin resistance, (3) body mass index, and (4) blood pressure[12].

Nuts enjoy a deserved reputation as health foods. A recent study used data from three longitudinal studies measuring 210,836 women who were free of cancer, heart disease, and stroke at baseline. Compared to women who never or almost never ate nuts, those who consumed five or more servings (at least five ounces) of nuts per week were 14 and 20 percent less likely to develop cardiovascular disease or coronary heart disease, respectively. We may reduce our risk of cardiovascular disease if we eat a serving of nuts every day[13].

Several studies link dietary fiber with reduced risk of ischemic heart disease (recurring chest pain from the heart not getting enough oxygen) and stroke in middle-aged persons. Does this protective effect extend to elderly persons, the fastest-growing segment of the U.S. population? Researchers used data from 3,588 participants in the Cardiovascular Health Study, a longitudinal cohort study of persons aged 65 years or older at baseline and followed for an average nine years. Participants with the highest level of cereal fiber intake (29 grams per day) had a 21 percent lower risk of new cardiovascular disease compared to those with the lowest level of fiber intake (5 grams per day). Older persons who increase their consumption of insoluble cereal fiber may reduce their risk of cardiovascular disease[14].

A systematic review and meta-analysis of 22 longitudinal studies revealed that higher total dietary fiber intake predicted lower risk of cardiovascular disease and coronary heart disease. Specifically, for each additional 7 grams of total fiber eaten each day, the risk declined by 9 percent. Thus, compared to a typical American who eats 14 grams of fiber per day, a person who eats 28 grams of fiber per day (similar to what health authorities recommend) would cut her risk of cardiovascular disease and coronary heart disease by 18 percent[15].

Researchers used data from several National Health and Nutrition Examination Surveys (1988-1994; 1999-2014; 2005-2010) to examine the association between added sugar (as a percent of dietary calories) and cardiovascular disease mortality. Most adults (71 percent) in the study consumed more than 10 percent of their daily calories from added sugar, and about 10 percent of the adults consumed more than 25 percent of their calories from added sugar. Compared to those in the lowest quintile of added sugar consumption (0 – 10 percent of calories as added sugar), persons in the highest quintile (greater than 21 percent) had double the risk of dying from cardiovascular disease.

The risk of cardiovascular mortality increased exponentially above 10 percent of daily calories from added sugar[16].

The Institute of Medicine (IOM) is a nonprofit organization that's part of the US National Academy of Sciences. The IOM operates separately from the government to provide evidence-based research and recommendations for public health and science policy. In 2005, the IOM recommended that calories from added sugar should be less than 25 percent of total calories, but this recommendation was not based on health considerations. The above study that used data from the National Health and Nutrition Examination Survey supported the World Health Organization's recommendation to limit intake of added sugar to 10 percent of daily calories based on health considerations.

Better blood sugar control

A recent meta-analysis included 15 studies that evaluated the effectiveness of a high-fiber diet for controlling blood sugar in type 2 diabetic subjects. Overall, fiber supplementation lowered fasting blood glucose by a clinically significant 15.32 mg/dL and HbA1c by a cynically meaningful 0.3 percentage points. HbA1c is a protein in the blood that shows average blood sugar levels over the previous 2-3 months. HbA1c levels above 6.5 percent signify type 2 diabetes. Incorporating more fiber in our diet can help control our blood sugar, whether we're diabetic or not[17].

Type 2 diabetes, which reflects higher than normal blood sugar, occurs in relatively low numbers in people following a vegan or vegetarian diet. Does a vegan diet help keep blood sugar at healthy levels comparable to the diet recommended by the American Diabetes Association (ADA)? To find out, researchers conducted a randomized controlled trial with 99 participants who followed either a vegan diet or the ADA diet. The vegan diet emphasized low fat (10 percent) and mostly complex carbohydrates (75 percent). The primary vegan foods included vegetables, fruits, grains, and legumes, with no meat or dairy and no added fats. The vegan diet emphasized low-glycemic index foods (slower-acting "good" carbs), such as beans and green vegetables. Quantities of food for the vegan diet were unlimited. The ADA diet included more protein (15–20 percent), less carbohydrates (60–70 percent), and more fat (10–15 percent) than the vegan diet. Food quantities for the ADA diet were limited.

Both the vegan diet and the ADA diet reduced blood levels of HbA1c, but the vegan diet led to greater reduction. On average, members of both diet groups lost weight, but members of the vegan group did so in spite of no limits on quantities of food eaten. Forty-three percent of the vegan diet group reduced their diabetes medications, compared to only 26 percent for the ADA diet group. While both diets improved blood sugar levels in diabetic persons, those on the vegan diet showed more improvement[18]. Some aspect(s) of a vegan diet appear to help keep blood sugar under control.

Reduced risk of diabetes

Both insoluble and soluble dietary fiber are associated with reduced weight gain and reduced inflammation, both of which appear to help regulate body weight. However, only insoluble dietary fiber, primarily from whole grains and bran, is associated with a reduced risk of diabetes in longitudinal studies[19].

The previously mentioned randomized PREDIMED trial by Spanish researchers found that the incidence of type 2 diabetes declined by 52 percent for those on the Mediterranean diets plus extra-virgin olive oil or mixed nuts combined, compared to those on the nominally low-fat diet. Notably, the reduced risk of diabetes occurred without a significant reduction in body weight[20].

Reduced risk of Alzheimer's disease

Foods do not affect our body independently of each other, because we commonly eat certain foods together or close together in time. In addition, studying the effects of one type of food at a time requires many studies to gather enough data to confidently state which specific foods best support our health and well-being. An alternative to studying the effects of one type of food at a time is studying combinations of foods that people might routinely eat. Researchers in New York employed this approach by investigating which food combinations might be associated with the risk of Alzheimer's disease. Researchers recruited 2,148 subjects who were followed for four years as part of the Washington Heights-Inwood Columbia Aging Project. Of the seven diet profiles developed by the researchers, only one predicted lower risk of Alzheimer's disease. Healthy foods in that diet profile included salad dressing, nuts, fish, tomatoes, poultry, cruciferous vegetables, fruits, and dark, leafy green vegetables. Unhealthy foods in that diet profile included high-fat dairy products, red meat, organ meat, and butter. Compared to the subjects whose diet fell in the lowest one-third of adherence to the healthy aspects of that diet profile, subjects whose diet fell in the highest one-third had a 38 percent lower risk of Alzheimer's disease. Generally speaking, the healthy diet profile resembled a Mediterranean diet[21].

Reduced risk of cancer

Eating lots of allium vegetables—garlic, onions, leeks, scallions, chives—predicts a reduced risk of prostate cancer. A study of 238 Chinese men who daily consumed more than 10 grams of allium vegetables (equivalent to about 1/8 cup of chopped onion) had a 58 percent lower risk of prostate cancer than men who consumed 2.2 grams of allium vegetables per day. Of the allium vegetables studied, scallions were linked to the greatest reduction in prostate cancer risk.

Men who ate more than 2.14 grams of scallions per day had a risk of prostate cancer that was 70 percent lower than that of men who ate no scallions. The reduction in risk of prostate cancer was greater for localized as opposed to advanced cancer[22].

The World Cancer Research Fund/American Institute for Cancer Research published its Second Expert Report *Food, Nutrition, Physical Activity and the Prevention of Cancer: A Global Perspective* in 2007. A recent study updated the report to reflect new research[23]. Evidence suggests that foods high in dietary fiber—especially whole grains, whole-grain cereals, and fruit—protect against colorectal cancer. Consumption of red meat, processed meat, and alcohol, as well as excess abdominal fat, are convincing causes of colorectal cancer. Garlic, milk, and calcium probably protect against colorectal cancer. Overall, the updated report concluded that food serves important roles in either preventing or causing colorectal cancer.

Improved cognitive function and brain health

Recent advances in imaging allow researchers to assess aspects of brain function relative to certain nutrients. In a study of 293 participants aged 65 or older and free of chronic cognitive problems, researchers periodically evaluated their cognitive function relative to serum nutrient biomarkers (substances used to indicate a disease or physiological state) until death. Two nutrient biomarker patterns predicted higher cognitive function and brain volume: pattern 1 included high levels of vitamins B1, B2, B6, B9, and B12, plus vitamins C, D, and E; pattern 2 included high levels of omega-3 fatty acids. The favorable effects of high levels of antioxidant vitamins and omega-3 fatty acids suggest that eating lots of dark green leafy and cruciferous vegetables, cold water fish, and fruits might promote cognitive function and brain health[24].

A recent literature review found that a Mediterranean diet can provide cognitive benefits and is certainly more healthful than the standard American diet[25]. Another recent trial confirmed that a Mediterranean diet (supplemented with additional extra-virgin olive oil or mixed nuts) predicted improved cognitive performance, perhaps due to abundant antioxidants and anti-inflammatory chemicals[26].

Reduced risk of cognitive decline

Strict adherence to a Mediterranean diet predicts not only better cognitive function but also slower rates of cognitive decline and a lower risk of Alzheimer's disease[25]. In two large multinational randomized trials with men and women age 55 and older that ran over five and six years respectively, the risk of developing cognitive impairment declined as the degree of healthy eating improved. Compared to those in the lowest quintile of healthy eating, those in the highest quintile had a 24 percent lower risk of exhibiting cognitive decline. If we *Eat Better,* our brains may work better over the long term[27].

A prospective study that was part of the Memory and Aging Project at the Rush Medical Center included 960 participants aged 58 to 99 years. Researchers investigated the relationship between green leafy vegetable consumption and the intake of select nutrients and phytochemicals—including vitamin K, lutein, beta-carotene, nitrate, folate, kaempferol, and alpha-tocopherol—with cognitive decline. Higher intakes of each of the nutrients and phytochemicals (except for beta-carotene) were individually associated with slower cognitive decline. After five years, compared to participants in the lowest quintile of green leafy vegetable consumption, participants in the highest quintile of green leafy vegetable consumption reduced their rate of cognitive decline, equating to being 11 years younger.

Wow! Continued consumption of the standard American diet by aging U.S. baby boomers could lead to huge increases in cognitive decline. But eating lots of kale, collard greens, spinach, Swiss chard, and other leafy greens might help maintain greater cognitive function later in life[28].

Improved microbiome health

There's been a lot of buzz lately about the human microbiome: the microbial, mostly bacterial, inhabitants our digestive tract, particularly the large intestine. With its stunning biological and biochemical complexity, the microbiome is sometimes called the second brain, reflecting the degree of control that it appears to exert over the entire body. For example, a simplified microbiome is linked to major health problems as noted below. Unsurprisingly, the food we eat greatly affects the composition and function of our microbiome.

Justin and Erica Sonnenburg, a husband-and-wife team of microbiology researchers at Stanford, propose a radical rethinking of the way we regard germs. Most of us regard microbes as bad, except for a few species that ferment malt into beer, milk into yogurt, or cabbage into kimchi. The Sonnenburgs make a compelling case that the three trillion microbial residents in our intestines provide a host of essential services without which we couldn't survive. In spite of the microbiome's critical role, many people aren't aware that it exists or perhaps take it for granted. Our ignorance and indifference wouldn't be an issue if the foods we Americans typically eat, along with our penchant for indiscriminately killing bacteria with antibiotics, didn't hammer our bacterial brethren. Our standard American diet—often highly processed, over-sweetened, calorie-dense, nutrient poor, stripped of fiber, and sanitized—is antithetical to a healthy gut because it reduces the bacterial diversity of our microbiome. Reduced microbial diversity is linked to a number of ills, including obesity, allergy, asthma, celiac disease, colonic inflammation, and frailty. The basic message: A happy microbiome promotes our health, but eating poor-quality food leads us in the wrong direction. The Sonnenburgs recommend the following:

Ways to Support a Healthy Microbiome

- Minimize consumption of added sugars and fruit juices.

- Ramp up consumption of veggies, fruits, and whole grains (preferably unmilled whole grains like old-fashioned rolled oats, brown rice, quinoa or wheat berries) to provide fiber that feeds the microbiome.

- Eat fermented foods, such as plain low-fat yogurt, tempeh, and kimchi, to increase microbiome diversity[29].

Reduced body fat

A recent study at the Mayo Clinic sought to determine whether excess body fat and reduced physical activity, rather than age itself, predict insulin sensitivity (the ability of insulin to help move blood glucose into cells). Researchers found that age was not a major independent predictor of insulin sensitivity when accounting for excess body fat. On the other hand, higher body fat independently predicted reduced insulin sensitivity. Therefore, eating foods that help prevent weight gain, along with participating regularly in aerobic exercise, will likely maintain insulin sensitivity and reduce the risk of type 2 diabetes with advancing age[30].

Poor Outcomes Linked to Failing to *Eat Better*

Unfortunately, failing to *Eat Better* may contribute to a host of serious chronic diseases and major markers of ill health. This section looks at seven negative outcomes that we want to avoid.

Bad Outcomes Linked to Failing to *Eat Better*

- Metabolic syndrome
- Type 2 diabetes
- Visceral fat deposition
- Hypertension
- Increased risk of premature death
- Obesity
- Osteoporosis

Metabolic syndrome

Metabolic syndrome is a cluster of symptoms—high blood pressure, high blood sugar, unhealthy cholesterol levels, and excess abdominal fat—that predict higher risks of heart disease, stroke, type 2 diabetes, and other health problems. Between 1996 and 2006, some 68 million Americans—25 percent of us—exhibited metabolic syndrome[31]. Eating better foods, especially those with a low-glycemic index and low-glycemic load, along with *Keep Moving*, can help prevent this undesirable outcome[32]. According to the World Health Organization, *insulin resistance is the principle cause of metabolic syndrome*. The standard American diet, with its emphasis on sugar, starch, and processed foods, plays a major role in increasing insulin resistance and, therefore, metabolic syndrome[33].

Glycemic Index and Glycemic Load

Glycemic index (GI) ranks foods from 0 to 100 according to how much they increase blood glucose levels. Carbs with a low GI (55 or less) are more slowly digested, absorbed, and metabolized, causing a lower and slower rise in blood glucose and insulin levels. Glycemic load (GL) is the product of GI and portion size. The GL is a better measure of how much a serving of carrots will elevate blood sugar (a little) compared to a serving of chocolate chip cookies (a lot). More healthful foods tend to have lower GI and GL values.

Researchers investigated the links between fiber and health markers using data from the 1999–2010 National Health and Nutrition Evaluation Survey (NHANES), a nationally representative, cross-sectional sample of the U.S. non-institutionalized civilian population. Mean dietary fiber intake was 16.2 grams per day for the sample of 23,168 subjects. From 1999 to 2010, fiber intake increased by an average of 1.3 grams per person per day, but fell below recommended levels during all 12 years of the survey. Compared to participants in the lowest quintile of fiber intake, subjects in the highest quintile had a statistically significant lower risk of metabolic syndrome (22 percent), inflammation (34 percent), and obesity (23 percent). In spite of the demonstrated health benefits of eating more fiber, Americans continue to consume far less fiber than recommended[34]. For specific recommendations, see the section "Eat More of These" later in this chapter.

Type 2 diabetes

The prevalence of type 2 diabetes in the U.S. and worldwide increased greatly over the past several decades. But this sad story has a platinum lining: Type 2 diabetes is almost entirely preventable by adopting healthy lifestyle choices. Plus, recent research shows that type 2 diabetes is reversible in many people within four years of diagnosis[35].

The average American gained a lot of weight over the past few decades. Could an increase in body fat account for the observed, simultaneous rise in diabetes? Researchers using data from NHANES found that the prevalence of diabetes rose from 7.4 percent to 12.3 percent between 1990 and 2015, a rise of 66 percent. Increase in body fat accounted for 72 percent of the rise in diabetes for both men and women. Higher food consumption (mostly sugars and starches) by Americans from 1990 to the present likely explains much of this increase in body fat. If we *Eat Better*, we'll be less likely to gain weight and develop diabetes[36].

Sugar intake, independent of obesity, is associated with the prevalence of type 2 diabetes. Data from 175 countries were used to test for associations between sugar availability and prevalence of diabetes. Researchers found that for every increase of 150 calories in daily sugar consumption (equivalent to a 12-ounce can of soft drink), the prevalence of diabetes increased by 1.1 percent, after controlling for a host of potential confounding factors. The more sugar we eat, the higher our risk of diabetes[37].

High consumption of sugar predicts greater incidence of non-alcoholic fatty liver disease (NAFLD), which affects about one-quarter of Americans. NALFD is a risk factor for type 2 diabetes and cardiovascular disease. Thus, high consumption of sugar can diminish overall health. Researchers in Europe conducted a controlled study in which 16 subjects consumed an extra 1,000 calories per day from candy and sweetened drinks for three weeks. During this time, body weight increased by an average of two percent; body mass index, waist and hip circumference, and abdominal subcutaneous fat all increased by three percent; intra-abdominal fat increased by five percent; and liver fat increased by 27 percent. After the initial three-week phase, the subjects were counseled to eat a more healthful diet to lose the weight they gained during the three weeks of overeating. Subsequently, the subjects lost four percent of their body weight and 25 percent of their liver fat. Thus, short-term overconsumption of sugar led to rapid increase in liver fat (27 percent), which was 13.5 times greater than the increase in body weight (2 percent). Cutting back on added sugar might reduce our risk of fatty liver disease, type 2 diabetes, and other maladies[38].

Other researchers used data from 70,842 subjects in the Nurses' Health Study and 40,787 subjects in the Health Professional Follow-up Study to evaluate the association between fried food consumption and new cases of both type 2 diabetes and coronary artery disease. Compared to subjects who ate fried food once a week or less, people who ate fried foods 1-3 times, 4-6 times, or 7 or more times per week had 15, 39, and 55 percent higher risk, respectively, of type 2 diabetes, regardless of confounding factors. Risks were generally higher for fried foods consumed away from home rather than at home[39].

Visceral fat deposition

While researchers commonly cite obesity as a cause of metabolic syndrome, obese individuals may exhibit no symptoms, while non-obese individuals may display one or more. Thus, obesity more likely serves as a marker rather than a cause of metabolic syndrome. The location of body fat, especially in the liver and pancreas, may be more important than its total bodily amount. According to British diabetes researcher Roy Taylor, prolonged caloric excess leads to fat deposition in the liver and subsequent fat deposition in the pancreas. Fat in the pancreas inhibits insulin secretion after meals, leading to elevated blood sugar and type 2 diabetes[35].

Hypertension

During the late 1990s, research showed that the so-called Dietary Approaches to Stop Hypertension (DASH) diet lowered blood pressure. This diet featured fruits, vegetables, and low-fat dairy products, low saturated fat, and low total fat. A follow-up study modified the DASH diet with higher levels of protein and monounsaturated fats (abundant in olive oil). Compared to the original DASH diet, the modified DASH diet reduced cardiovascular risk, triglycerides, and blood pressure. Both the DASH and the modified DASH diets reduced total cholesterol and LDL-cholesterol (the "bad" kind). Reducing carb intake (especially sugars and starches) and increasing either protein or monounsaturated fats improved the effectiveness of the DASH diet in reducing blood pressure and the risk of cardiovascular disease[40].

Does a vegetarian diet predict lower blood pressure? A recent meta-analysis of 39 studies found that, compared to omnivorous diets, vegetarian diets predicted significantly reduced systolic and diastolic blood pressures of 4.8 and 2.2 mm Hg, respectively. To put these numbers in context, a 5 mm reduction in systolic blood pressure predicts a 7 percent reduction in death due to all causes, a 9 percent reduction in coronary heart disease, and a 4 percent reduction in stroke. This meta-analysis suggests that one or more aspects of a vegetarian diet can lead to lower blood pressure and reduced risk of hypertension[41].

Increased risk of premature death

Cardiovascular disease, which includes coronary heart disease, heart attack, and stroke, is the number-one killer in the U.S. Thus, identifying the causes and their relative contributions to overall risk of premature death could inform effective preventive measures. Higher consumption of sugar- and artificially sweetened beverages predicts higher cardiometabolic risk. But does consumption of artificially sweetened beverages predict the risk of stroke or dementia? The Framingham, Massachusetts, Heart Study Offspring Study began in 1971, following 5,124 volunteers for an average of 10 years. Compared to participants who didn't consume any artificially sweetened beverages, those who consumed one or more artificially sweetened drinks per week had a 196 percent higher risk of ischemic stroke and 189 percent higher risk of Alzheimer's disease during follow-up[42]. Artificially sweetened beverages may not be a benign alternative to sugar-sweetened beverages. A new study confirmed that higher consumption of sugar-sweetened beverages, but not artificially sweetened beverages, predicted higher risk of premature death[43].

Researchers reviewed longitudinal studies and randomized trials to calculate the risk of death of cardiovascular disease patients. Those who met all of the following dietary recommendations had a 454 percent lower risk of death. This reduction in risk exceeds that of commonly prescribed cardioprotective drugs, such as low-dose aspirin, statins, and beta blockers.

- Limit intake of saturated fat to less than 10 percent of energy. Assuming a caloric intake of 2,000 calories per day, this equates to 22 grams of saturated fat per day or the amount of saturated fat in a little more than one quart of reduced-fat milk.

- Eat oily fish at least once a week.

- Eat at least five servings of vegetables and fruits per day.

- Eat more than 28 grams of fiber from unrefined whole grains, legumes, and nuts per day.

- Reduce salt intake to less than one-half teaspoon per day[44].

Altering food consumption as outlined above, along with exercising regularly, not smoking, and maintaining a healthy body weight may prevent most coronary heart disease in the U.S.[45] Now imagine what might happen if we adopted more of the nine lifestyle choices that this book champions!

Researchers in Sweden recently conducted a prospective study of survival over a 15-year period in relation to meat consumption in a group of 74,645 middle-aged adults. High consumption (more than 100 grams or about 3.5 ounces per day) of processed red meat predicted shorter survival. High and moderate (about 50 grams per day) consumption of unprocessed red meat predicted shorter survival, but only when accompanied by a high intake of processed meat. Consumption of unprocessed red meat alone did not predict survival over a 15-year period. Thus, carefully consider studies that combine unprocessed and processed red meat into one category. Any adverse effect of red meat consumption in such studies might reflect the impact of processed rather than unprocessed red meat[46].

Unprocessed and processed meats appear to have different effects on human health. A study of 448,568 participants in the European Investigation into Cancer and Nutrition included 10 countries with varied diets. Unprocessed red meat consumption was not significantly associated with all-cause mortality, cardiovascular disease, or cancer, while higher consumption of processed red meat was significantly associated with a higher risk of premature death. Notably, this study does not support the notion that eating low amounts of unprocessed red meat is bad for your health[47].

Researchers developed a risk model using data from NHANES (1999-2002, 2009-2012). The model estimated associations of 10 dietary factors with cardiometabolic diseases from meta-analyses of prospective studies and clinical trials. The dietary factors included fruits, vegetables, nuts/seeds, whole grains, unprocessed red meats, processed meats, sugar-sweetened beverages, polyunsaturated fats, seafood omega-3 fats, and sodium (in table salt). Of the 702,308 cardiometabolic deaths that occurred in the U.S. in 2012, an estimated 45 percent were associated with suboptimal intakes (either too low or too high) of these 10 dietary factors. Excessive sodium consumption (from table salt) accounted for the largest proportion of deaths (9.5 percent), followed by low nuts/seeds consumption (8.5 percent), high processed meats (8.2 percent), low seafood omega-3 fats (7.8 percent), low vegetables (7.3 percent), low fruits (7.5 percent), and high sugar-sweetened beverages (7.4 percent). Thus, it appears that reducing levels of sodium, processed meats, and sugar, while eating more nuts, seeds, vegetables, fruits, and omega-3 fats in seafood would likely reduce our risk of death from cardiometabolic diseases[48].

Obesity

Obesity and being overweight are increasingly prevalent in both developed and developing countries. Eating excessive amounts of poor-quality foods is the most common explanation for the overall rise in girth. Insufficient movement, commonly termed "lack of exercise" or "a sedentary lifestyle," is also cited as a contributor.

Since 1980, the number of Americans classified as obese (body mass index of 30 or more) doubled. Researchers at the University of North Carolina studying this surge in obesity found that Americans consumed an average of 570 more calories a day from 1977–1978 to 2003–2006. Beverages and solid foods accounted for 203 and 367 additional calories, respectively. Moreover, the average number of daily eating opportunities increased from 3.8 to 4.9 over that period; portion sizes for both beverages and solid food also increased. Thus, eating less often and reducing portion size might help reduce the risk of obesity[49].

The U.S. farm bills in the 1970s may have contributed to the rise in obesity among Americans. Starting around 1977, these farm bills led to increased food production, bigger portion sizes, accelerated food marketing, and greater affordability of energy-dense (aka higher-calorie) foods, along with the widespread introduction of high-fructose corn syrup as a sweetener[50].

What Promotes Overeating?

Eating palatable but low-cost, nutrient-poor, high-calorie foods and beverages enhances our sensitivity to cues related to food rewards, thus leading to overeating. Being in a negative mood can also promote overeating, as can exposure to chronic stress. Adverse early-life experiences may exacerbate stress-induced overeating later in life. An effective tactic to reduce overeating is to avoid buying foods that are highly appealing but contain minimal nutritional value. Such foods provide cues that promote overeating[51]. Leave such foods at the grocery store.

Reducing sugar consumption can promote weight loss. Robert Lustig, a researcher who specializes in sugar, and his colleagues recruited 43 Los Angeles–area Latino and African American obese children who also exhibited symptoms of metabolic syndrome. During a 10-day study, sugar from the children's diets was replaced, calorie for calorie, with starches. (Starches were used to maintain the same level of calories in the kids' diets, not because of starches' health value.) After 10 days, the children lost an average of one pound of body weight. Blood markers (triglycerides, LDL cholesterol, glucose tolerance, and high blood fats) improved significantly, as did diastolic blood pressure. Minimizing intake of added sugar—without reducing total calories—led to short-term weight loss and clinically meaningful improvements in obesity and biomarkers for type 2 diabetes[52].

Strong evidence suggests that high dietary fiber intake protects against overweight and obesity. A recent review evaluated randomized trials of soluble fiber supplementation in overweight and obese adults with respect to weight, body fat, and metabolism. Based on 12 studies, supplementation with soluble fiber led to significant reductions in body mass index (0.84 units) and body weight (5.54 pounds), compared to placebo controls. Body fat, fasting glucose, and fasting insulin also declined. Eating more soluble fiber in the form of non-starchy vegetables, fruits, and oats/oatmeal/oat bran may improve our health by helping keep our body weight under control and improving blood glucose metabolism[53].

Osteoporosis

Osteoporosis is a major public health problem characterized by weak, brittle bones. This condition, especially common in postmenopausal women, greatly increases the risk of hip, spine, and forearm fractures. Happily, osteoporosis can be prevented (or the lifetime risk greatly reduced) with healthy lifestyle choices, ideally begun during adolescence.

For the general population, recommendations from the National Osteoporosis Foundation include adequate intake of calcium and vitamin D, lifelong participation in weight-bearing and muscle-strengthening exercise, no tobacco use, no (or limited) alcohol consumption, and treatment of risk factors for falling. Aside from supplements, dairy products are the chief sources of calcium and vitamin D for most Americans, while sun exposure can provide additional vitamin D[54].

Studies show that high fruit and vegetable consumption predicts improved bone mineral density. Animal studies reveal that dried plums (prunes) prevent bone loss in laboratory rats. A three-month study with postmenopausal women who consumed 100 grams (3.6 ounces) of dried plums showed improved markers of bone regeneration. A one-year randomized trial included 160 postmenopausal women who ate either 100 grams of dried plums or 75 grams (2.7 ounces) of dried apples daily. Dried plums led to significantly increased bone density in the forearm and spine compared to dried apples. In addition, dried plums reduced levels of two bone mineral depletion markers[55].

Eat More of These

In *The 150 Healthiest Foods on Earth*, nutrition expert Jonny Bowden[56] provides an evenhanded and evidence-based treatment of the complex issue of what we eat. After reading his book, I decided to emphasize Bowden's list of "super foods" (see sidebar), which includes an even more rarefied list of his favorite food choices, what he calls "all-star veggies." I suggest making these super foods the centerpiece of your eating. These days, Bowden's super foods account for about three-quarters (on a food weight basis) of what my wife and I eat. The other quarter comes largely from other items in his list of 150 healthiest foods.

Green leafy vegetables

Jonny Bowden lists dandelion, kale, spinach, Swiss chard, collard greens, and watercress as super foods. Arugula is another green leafy veggie that works well in salads. I recommend replacing iceberg lettuce (which contains minimal nutrients) with a more nutritious variety (such as Romaine or red leaf) or going with spinach or arugula. Green leafy vegetables are easy to grow in most gardens, even those that don't receive a lot of sun.

Colorful, non-starchy vegetables

Colorful vegetables, aside from the green leafy kind, contain an array of vitamins and other compounds that appear to have health-enhancing properties. For example, cruciferous veggies contain substances called glucosinolates. Some of the break-down products of glucosinolates, including sulforaphane, protect against cancer[57]. Cruciferous veggies include kale, broccoli, Brussels sprouts, cabbage, cauliflower, collards, and bok choy. Other candidates include green beans, zucchini, summer squash, eggplant, carrots, and tomatoes. Winter squash, potatoes, sweet potatoes, and yams are starchy vegetables, although they have lots of nutritional value.

Jonny Bowden's Super Foods

Vegetables: beets, broccoli, Brussels sprouts, cabbage, carrots, dandelion, mushrooms, onions, spinach, Swiss chard, watercress

Grains: oatmeal, quinoa

Beans: lentils

Fruits: avocados, blueberries, cherries, coconut, guava, kiwifruit, strawberries

Nuts, seeds, and nut butters: almonds (and almond butter), pecans, walnuts

Soy foods: natto (fermented soybeans)

Dairy: butter (organic, from pasture-fed cows), raw organic milk, yogurt

Meat, poultry, eggs, fish and seafood: sardines, wild Alaska salmon

Specialty foods: bee pollen, green foods and drinks, kimchi, sauerkraut, sea veggies, sprouts, whey protein powder

Beverages: fresh vegetable juice, pomegranate juice, tea, water

Spices: cinnamon, garlic, ginger, oregano, turmeric

Oils: coconut oil, extra virgin olive oil, flaxseed oil, macadamia nut oil

Fiber

Dietary fiber refers to carbohydrates the body cannot digest or absorb. Unlike other food components, it passes relatively intact through the stomach, small intestine, colon, and out of the body. Fiber is found primarily in whole grains, fruits, vegetables, and legumes. There are two main types of fiber, both beneficial to health: soluble and insoluble. Soluble fiber (found mostly in fruits, veggies, and oats) dissolves in water and can help lower blood glucose and cholesterol levels. Insoluble fiber (found mostly in grains such as wheat) does not dissolve in water. It can help move food through the digestive system, thereby promoting regularity and preventing constipation.

Most Americans consume far too little dietary fiber. The typical American adult eats 14-16 grams of fiber per day. High-fiber diets include intakes of at least 28 and 38 grams per day for women and men, respectively[58]. Increasing our intake of dietary fiber (see sidebar) would likely provide a variety of health benefits. Interestingly, contemporary African hunter-gatherers consume huge amounts of fiber (80–150 grams daily) and exhibit little to no cardiovascular disease, type 2 diabetes, or obesity[59].

How Much Fiber Should We Eat Every Day?

The Institute of Medicine recommends the following minimum daily intake levels for total fiber:

- Men aged 19-50 years: 38 grams
- Men over age 50: 30 grams
- Women aged 19-50 years: 25 grams
- Women over age 50: 21 grams

Fruits

Fruits contain vitamins, antioxidants, and an array of other nutrients that have protective benefits. Health experts recommend we eat one or more servings of fruit daily. Here's how to make better fruit choices:

- Eat the whole fruit (minus the rind, core, etc.) instead of fruit juice. The whole fruit contains fiber that's often not found in the juice, and it takes longer to chew and digest, thereby reducing the subsequent blood-sugar spike.

- Focus on fruits with a lower glycemic load, meaning those containing less natural sugar. Berries, such as blueberries, usually have lower glycemic loads. Dried fruits (raisins, prunes, dates) and tropical fruits (bananas, pineapples, mangos) have higher glycemic loads.
  (See *https://extension.oregonstate.edu/sites/default/files/documents/1/glycemicindex.pdf for a list of common foods and their glycemic loads.*)

- Even though there's no agreed-upon upper limit for consumption of sugar that naturally occurs in fruits, I suggest not eating massive quantities of fruits. In peach season in Colorado, I used to eat three to four mouth-watering peaches each day. That amounted to 39 to 52 grams of sugar. I've cut that to one peach per day (13 grams of sugar) that I savor for its scrumptious flavor. I usually eat blueberries, an orange, and an apple each day.

Nuts

Tree nuts include almonds, Brazil nuts, cashews, chestnuts, hazelnuts, macadamia nuts, pecans, and walnuts. Peanuts are not tree nuts (they grow in the soil) but are commonly lumped in the "nut" category. Some people are allergic to tree nuts or peanuts. If you aren't, tree nuts are excellent sources of protein and fiber.

Onions, garlic, and their relatives

Allium vegetables (onions, garlic, scallions, chives, leeks) are healthy staples of many Asian diets. Their many health benefits are thought to reflect their abundant sulfur-containing compounds. Plus, they give life to otherwise bland foods.

Olive oil

Olive oil, a key part of the Mediterranean diet, is rich in monounsaturated fat. I recommend buying extra-virgin, cold-pressed olive oil. Compared to polyunsaturated oils (such as corn oil), olive oil degrades less at high temperatures. Nevertheless, I minimize high cooking temperatures to reduce the risk of degrading olive oil and producing unhealthy chemicals. I sprinkle olive oil over steamed veggies to heighten their flavor.

Wild, cold water fish

The long-standing recommendation from the American Heart Association and others to eat less saturated fat prompted Americans to use polyunsaturated vegetable oils (including corn, sunflower, safflower, soybean, and cottonseed). These oils contain a high ratio of omega-6 to omega-3 fatty acids. Omega-6 fatty acids are essential, but can be harmful when consumed in excess. For most people, an omega-6 to omega-3 ratio of 4:1 is ideal. I use polyunsaturated oils sparingly, favoring monounsaturated olive oil, thereby reducing the amount of omega-6 fatty acids. Eating foods with abundant omega-3 fatty acids include wild-caught, cold water fish (salmon, halibut, sardines) can help bring the ratio back into the desirable range. So can eating grass-fed animal products (milk, cheese, meat).

Whole grains

Whole grains are literally whole intact seeds that haven't been milled into flour. They include brown rice, quinoa, buckwheat, barley, and millet. Old-fashioned rolled oats and cracked wheat come close to being whole grains. The nutritional value of whole grains arises in large part from the fiber and other complex carbohydrates, vitamins, and minerals they contain. Whole grains provide lots of indigestible fiber, which is linked to reduced risk of type 2 diabetes and other chronic diseases[58]. Because we digest whole grains slower than refined grains, their glycemic index values are lower. Lower glycemic index foods lead to lower post-meal blood sugar spikes compared to higher glycemic-index foods such as refined carbohydrates and sugar.

Eat Less of These

In spite of the current debate about which foods to avoid, researchers generally recommend eating less trans fats (partially hydrogenated vegetable oils), added sugar, refined grains, processed meat products, deep-fried food, and salt. If we reduce our consumption of them, we'll *Eat Better*.

Trans fats

In the 1950s, food manufacturers started adding trans fats to improve the consistency and shelf life of many processed foods, including snack foods, baked goods, and margarine. However, a wealth of evidence links trans fats with numerous health problems, including inflammation, increased risk of cardiovascular disease, and all-cause mortality[60]. Consequently, the U.S. Food and Drug Administration ruled trans fats unsafe to eat and officially outlawed them as additives in foods and restaurants in the U.S. as of 2018. Note that food products can have less than 0.5 grams of trans fat per serving without that being stated on the label.

Added sugar

The U.S. Department of Agriculture (USDA) keeps tabs on how much we eat each year. A 2008 report from the Economic Research Service of the USDA compared changes in the average per capita consumption of specific foods and food groups from 1970 to 2005[61]. Over this period, added sugar and sweetener availability (reflecting the amount of sugar produced in the U. S. and imported from other countries, not adjusted for losses due to spoilage) in America increased by 19 percent—for a total of 142 pounds per year. This increase largely reflects greater U. S. consumption of high-fructose corn syrup. Over the same period, daily food intake by Americans increased by an average of 150–300 calories, with about half of the increase coming from liquid calories, mainly sugar-sweetened beverages.

Recommended Limits of Added Sugar

In 2009, the American Heart Association[62] issued the following upper-limit guidelines for daily consumption of added sugar:

- Adult males: less than nine teaspoons or 36 grams (150 calories)
- Adult females: less than 5–6 teaspoons or 20 grams (100 calories)
- Children: less than three teaspoons or 12 grams (50 calories)

The rising tide of obesity and overweight mirrors the rise in consumption of added sugar. Nutritional experts generally advise cutting back on sodas, sports drinks, sweetened teas, and other beverages with lots of added sugar.

A 12-ounce can of Mountain Dew soda contains 46 grams of sugar. That corresponds to more than a two-day allowance of added sugar for women, and 28 percent more than a daily allowance for men. A 24-ounce can of Arizona Ice Tea contains 72 grams of added sugar. The can contains three servings, but how many people drink just one-third of a can in one sitting?

Mounting evidence suggests that typical U.S. consumption levels of added sugar increase the risk of premature mortality and several chronic diseases, including metabolic syndrome conditions[63]. Gary Taubes, in his meticulously documented book, *The Case Against Sugar*, argues that added sugar is the most likely cause for the increase in chronic diseases associated with Western civilization. These conditions include type 2 diabetes, obesity, and gout. Taubes concedes that the evidence isn't iron-clad (and may never be due to practical constraints), but why not err on the side of caution and adopt a prudent approach and minimize consumption of added sugar?

Refined grains

Refined grains include flour and products made from flour: most breads, bagels, cookies, crackers, cakes, and many snacks. These products often contain a lot of added sugar and lack nutritionally valuable ingredients. Numerous products, such as bread, tout their nutritional value because they contain whole grains. But many products labeled "whole grain" have a considerable amount of white flour. Bread products may contain only small amounts of whole-wheat flour (hence the advertising phrase "made with whole grains").

Read the list of ingredients to see where white flour, also called wheat flour (which is not the same as *whole-wheat flour*), falls. If white flour appears first, the product contains mostly white flour.

So why knock refined grains? There are several reasons. First, white flour has been stripped of the bran and the germ, so it has little nutrient value unless it is fortified. Even then, not all of the lost nutrition is replaced. Second, white flour is readily digested (by most people), which can create sharp spikes in blood sugar. Milling increases the digestibility of the grain, typically increasing its glycemic index. Thus, white flour has a relatively high glycemic index and high glycemic load. Prolonged consumption of high-glycemic foods increases the risk of type 2 diabetes and other maladies. (People with gluten sensitivity need to stay away from wheat and rye. And, while oats don't contain gluten, oats may become contaminated with gluten if housed in facilities that also store gluten-containing grains.)

I suggest going easy on refined grains in their many forms, especially white flour. Tasty breads, chips, crackers, and cakes are often empty calories, and it's easy to overeat them. How about buying them infrequently, buying them in small packages, or leaving them at the store altogether?

Processed meat products

When evaluating effects on health, it's useful to distinguish between processed and unprocessed red meat. Processed meats include sausage, hot dogs, salami, ham, and liver paté. Unprocessed meats refer to fresh cuts (such as steaks and roasts) and ground beef. Moderate to high consumption of processed meat products predicts an increased risk of mortality, cardiovascular disease, prostate cancer, and colorectal cancer.

Deep-fried foods

Frying is a common way to prepare food for eating. French fries, fried chicken, fried eggs: these are favorites for many Americans. Although the science underlying the health effects of fried foods is mixed, most findings show that fried foods—especially deep-fried foods—don't support good health. In spite of the conflicting evidence about the extent to which fried foods contribute to ill health, studies suggest that the prudent path is to reduce their intake to less than four times per week[64]. The following tips can reduce the health risks of fried foods:

- Pan-fry rather than deep-fry.
- Fry at relatively low temperatures as opposed to high temperatures.
- Use olive or coconut oil rather than polyunsaturated oils.
- Don't eat foods fried in reused oils, as in fast-food outlets.

Salt

Physicians have long urged their patients to limit their intake of salt to reduce the risk of heart disease and stroke. Sodium plays several essential roles in the body and occurs naturally in many foods. Much of the salt we eat is added to foods we buy, and many of us add salt while cooking or eating to season our food. While there is no consensus as to whether Americans eat too much salt[65], the Institute of Medicine recommends salt intakes between 1,500 and 2,300 mg per day. A quarter teaspoon of table salt contains 1,500 mg.

Over the years, I've lowered my consumption of salt by gradually using less and less of it. My taste buds are now accustomed to a low-salt diet. I rarely add salt to cooked food, and when I do, I use it sparingly.

Foods That Are Maybe Yes, Maybe No

Much of what we've been told about the effects of the foods we eat does not reflect sound science. This section covers selected foods—eggs, grass-fed animal products, and red meat—for which research is mixed. Some studies suggest that eating these foods predicts an increased risk of certain diseases, while other research does not. My understanding of current research suggests that consuming these foods in moderation is healthful.

Eggs

For many years, some nutritional experts have advised us to limit our consumption of eggs, or at least the yolks, because of their high cholesterol content. Actually, cholesterol is essential for life, especially for our brain. Our liver produces cholesterol, typically far more than we consume in our food[66]. Research shows that our bodies produce less cholesterol when we eat a lot of it[67].

This may account for the observation that eating two to three eggs per day over a long period of time predicts only a minor increase in serum cholesterol in, at most, the vast majority of Americans[68]. The Physician's Health Study did not detect a significant link between the consumption of one egg per day and the risk of cardiovascular disease. However, eating more than one egg a day predicted a significant 22 percent increase in the risk of all-cause mortality. Furthermore, diabetic participants who ate at least seven eggs per week had double the risk of all-cause mortality, compared to diabetics who ate less than one egg per week[69]. To further muddy the waters, a new study found that each 300 mg increase in daily cholesterol and each one-half of an egg intake predicted 17 and 6 percent increase in risks of cardiovascular disease, respectively[70].

Grass-fed animal products

Until about 1950, most of the beef eaten in the U.S. came from animals
raised in pastures on farms and ranches. Those cattle ate grass and
other green plants for their entire lives. They didn't spend their last
few months in feedlots, eating grains. Today, the vast majority of beef
comes from cattle that are fattened on grain in feedlots.

Loren Cordain and colleagues analyzed the fatty acids in various
pasture-raised ruminant animals (cattle, sheep, goats), along with
conventional (feedlot) and pasture-raised steers. They found that the
muscle of pasture-raised steers had 42 percent less total fat and 52
percent less saturated fat than feedlot steers. Data from the researchers
suggest that saturated fat in grass-fed and feedlot steers are similar
(see Table 2.1). In addition, pasture-raised steers had omega-6 to
omega-3 fatty acids ratios of 2.26:1. Feedlot steers had omega-6 to
omega-3 fatty acids ratios of 5.28:1. Evolutionary evidence favors
omega-6 to omega-3 fatty acid ratios between 1:1 and 4:1 for humans.
Early humans may have adapted to the omega-6 to omega-3 ratio
found in the wild mammals that generations of early humans ate. For
this and other reasons discussed below, it seems unlikely moderate
amounts of grass-fed animal products (meat, milk, cheese) promote
cardiovascular disease, in spite of the cholesterol and saturated fat
that these products contain[71].

Meat of grain-fed cattle has a very different nutrient profile than
that of grass-fed cattle or of contemporary wild mammals. The difference in nutritional profiles of grain-fed and grass-fed cattle in Table
2.1 tend to favor grass-fed over conventional beef.

Table 2.1. Characteristics of Grass-Fed and Conventional Meat[72]		
Characteristic	Grass-Fed	Conventional
Total fat	Lower	Higher
Saturated fat	Same	Same
Myristic and palmitic fatty acids (linked to higher risk of cardiovascular disease)	Lower	Higher
Omega-6: Omega-3 fatty acid ratio	Lower	Higher
Conjugated linoleic acid	Higher	Lower
Vitamins A and E	Higher	Lower
Glutathione	Higher	Lower

Meat of grain-fed cattle has a very different nutrient profile than that of grass-fed cattle or of contemporary wild mammals. The difference in nutritional profiles of grain-fed and grass-fed cattle in Table 2.1 indicates that modern beef comes from a whole different animal than those that existed just 70 years ago.

Red meat

If meat consumption is bad for our health, it follows that vegetarians would be healthier and live longer than nonvegetarians. Three studies from the United Kingdom indicate otherwise[73].

1. **The Healthy Food Shoppers Study** included 10,736 persons who were customers of health food shops, members of vegetarian societies, and readers of health-related magazines. The subjects—43 percent vegetarians and 57 percent nonvegetarians—were recruited from 1973 to 1979, with follow-up until 1997. During the follow-up period, the standardized mortality rate for *both* vegetarians and nonvegetarians was 41 percent lower than that of the entire United Kingdom.

2. **The Oxford Vegetarian Study** recruited 11,045 subjects from 1980 to 1984 through both the Vegetarian Society of the U.K. and news media. Nonvegetarian subjects were recruited by the vegetarian participants from among their friends and relatives. The entire group was followed until 2000. During the follow-up period, the standardized mortality rates for vegetarians and nonvegetarians were 51 percent and 54 percent, respectively. This difference was not statistically significant.

3. **The EPIC-Oxford Vegetarian Study** recruited adults over age 35 from general practice surgeries in the U.K. from 1993 to 1999, with follow-up until 2002. After five years of follow-up, the standardized mortality rates for vegetarians and nonvegetarians were 40 percent and 39 percent, respectively.

These studies suggest that vegetarians are much healthier than average U.K. citizens, but not because the vegetarians don't eat meat. These studies do not support the idea that red meat is bad for our health. Presumably, both vegetarians and their meat-eating friends adopt more healthy choices than the typical U.K. citizen, thus accounting for their lower mortality rate.

Red meat consumption has been associated with an increased risk of cardiovascular disease and cancer, but diet studies often don't distinguish between processed and unprocessed meats. A recent study used data from 1986 to 2010 to evaluate the relationship between meat consumption, diet quality, and risk of mortality. After 22 years of follow-up, both high unprocessed red meat consumption (eaten 44 times a month) and high processed meat consumption (eaten 29 times a month) were significantly associated with increased mortality. When multiple confounding factors were taken into account, the associations were no longer significant, suggesting that those who consumed lots of unprocessed red meat and/or processed meat tended to make unhealthy lifestyle choices, such as smoking. For men but not women, the risk of all-cause mortality declined as white meat consumption and healthy eating scores increased. The relationships between unprocessed and processed meat and measures of health appear to be more complicated than first imagined[74].

Dietary advice to limit red meat is intended to limit consumption of saturated fats. Two recent Canadian studies found that stearic acid, one the most common saturated fats in red meat, did not increase LDL ("bad") cholesterol levels. The authors argued that current Canadian diets reflect declines in the consumption of unprocessed or minimally processed foods (such as meat, milk, eggs, vegetables, nuts, and seeds) and increases in eating highly processed, ready-to-eat foods. The authors concluded that reducing unprocessed red meat consumption would have a much lower positive effect on diet quality and health compared to reducing salt and increasing the intake of vegetables, whole grains, fruits, nuts, and seeds[75].

Low-Fat or Low-Carb?

We don't have to look far to find blog posts and articles extolling the virtues of either a low-fat or low-carb approach to eating. Losing weight or maintaining weight loss is often the context. Yet the debate over low-carb or low-fat diets may miss the main point of *Eat Better*.

European researchers studied people who had lost at least eight percent of their body weight. The weight-losers were followed for 26 weeks to determine if certain diets would maintain the weight loss, compared to a control diet. The diets contained either: (1) high protein and high glycemic, (2) high protein and low glycemic, (3) low protein and high glycemic, or (4) low protein and low glycemic. The control diet followed the dietary guidelines of the country in which each subject lived.

Those who ate either of the two high-protein diets were more likely than those who ate either of the low-protein diets to achieve additional weight loss during the maintenance phase. Only participants in the low-protein and high-glycemic diet groups experienced significant weight regain. Modest increases in protein and low-glycemic index foods minimized weight regain or promoted further weight loss in overweight or obese patients following weight loss. Ready access to low-glycemic index foods (such as leafy greens and non-starchy veggies) and support from friends may have facilitated successful weight-loss maintenance[76].

If you're attempting to lose weight and keep it off, should you eat a low-fat or a low-carb diet? Maybe that's the wrong question. A recent clinical trial reported that both a healthy low-fat diet and a healthy low-carb diet led to similar weight loss (5.2 and 6.0 kg, respectively) over one year[77]. Here's what researchers included in the "healthy" diets:

- All participants were instructed to focus on whole, real foods prepared mostly at home, specifically vegetables, lean grass-fed and pasture-raised animal foods, and sustainably harvested fish. They were also advised to eliminate or minimize processed foods that contained added sugars, refined white flour, or trans fats. Participants were told to eat fresh, seasonal foods when possible and to request menu modifications when eating out, in keeping with their group's diet assignment.

- Participants in the healthy low-fat group were asked to reduce their consumption of edible oils, fatty meats, whole-fat dairy products, and nuts.

- Participants in the healthy low-carb group were encouraged to reduce consumption of cereals, grains, rice, starchy vegetables, and legumes.

Although participants were not instructed to limit calories, members of both diet groups did reduce their daily caloric intake, though the difference was not statistically significant. The big lesson from this study: Either a healthy low-fat or healthy low-carb diet would be fine to lose weight and keep it off. The key word is "healthy." In other words, *Eat Better*.

Mediterranean Diet

A Mediterranean-type diet appears to protect against a variety of ills, including metabolic syndrome symptoms. This diet typically features olive oil as a main source of fat and calories. Veggies, fruits, nuts, whole grains, yogurt, fish, legumes, and red wine are also prominent. Products derived from white flour (such as pasta) and processed foods are typically not part of a Mediterranean diet.

If a Mediterranean diet truly promotes health, it's impossible to say exactly what in this diet is responsible. Is it the olive oil? How about the emphasis on vegetables? Could it be the red wine? The minimal use of processed food?

Perhaps diet is not the leading cause of better health of people in Mediterranean countries. Dan Buettner, author of *The Blue Zones,* studied the diet and lifestyle habits of the residents of Ikaria. This Greek island in the Mediterranean Sea boasts an inordinately high proportion of centenarians. Buettner attributed their health and longevity to a suite of factors he calls "the Power 9 Principles". They include move naturally, purpose, downshift, eat until 80 percent full, eat mostly plants, drink wine at 5 p.m., find the right tribe, put loved ones first, and belong[78]. Sounds a lot like the nine healthy lifestyle choices, doesn't it? A Mediterranean-type diet is probably healthful, particularly compared to the standard American diet, but other lifestyle choices are also important.

Paleo Diet

Our ancient hunter-gatherer, pre-human and human ancestors adapted genetically to eating a diet consisting of wild plants and animals, namely lean meat, fruits, vegetables, and nuts. The genetic makeup of modern humans is not that different from our ancient ancestors. It follows, then, that eating foods that mimic those available to our ancestors would support our health and well-being.

If a Paleolithic-type diet is nutritionally superior to the standard American diet, then people who eat a Paleo diet should exhibit improved biochemical markers. To find out, San Francisco researchers studied six males and three females who were slightly overweight and sedentary, with an average age of 40 years. All the subjects ate their usual diets for three days, then over the next seven days ate a transitional diet with increasing amounts of potassium and fiber. For the next 10 days, the subjects ate a Paleo-type diet of lean meats, fruits, vegetables, nuts, and small amounts of honey. Cereal grains, dairy products, and legumes were excluded. On the Paleo diet, participants ate an average of 2,701 calories per day, roughly 329 more calories than their usual diets. At the end of the 10-day Paleo diet, eight of the nine subjects showed improved biochemical profiles. The Paleo diet led to significant, healthful reductions in blood fats (total cholesterol, LDL cholesterol, VLDL cholesterol, triglycerides), greater insulin sensitivity, lower fasting insulin/fasting glucose, and lower diastolic blood pressure. Thus, a Paleo-type diet may provide rapid and substantial health benefits, especially compared to the standard American diet[79].

Front-Load Daily Food Consumption

Shifting when we eat—especially high-calorie foods and protein—to earlier in the day may help us avoid weight gain, even if the amount and composition of what we eat doesn't change. In a study by Israeli researchers, overweight and obese women were randomly assigned to one of two weight-loss diets. Women in Diet 1 ate 50 percent of their daily calories at breakfast, 36 percent at lunch, and 14 percent at dinner. Women in Diet 2 ate 14 percent of their daily calories at breakfast, 36 percent at lunch, and 50 percent at dinner. Both diets had 1,400 calories per day. Subjects in Diet 1 achieved significantly greater weight loss as well as healthier blood chemistry (lower fasting glucose, insulin, insulin resistance), and experienced less hunger than the other women[80].

Skipping breakfast altogether to lose weight may be especially counterproductive. To the contrary, eating a big breakfast that's high in fat and protein may improve health. In another Israeli study, obese or overweight subjects aged 47 to 70 were randomly assigned to one of two diets. The Big Breakfast diet was rich in fat and protein and contained 33 percent of daily calories. The Small Breakfast diet was rich in carbohydrates and contained 12.5 percent of daily calories. Both diets had the same number of daily calories, which was 500 calories less than that required to maintain a stable weight.

Over three months, all the subjects consumed about 150–200 more calories per day than recommended. Yet subjects in the Big Breakfast group had significantly lower systolic blood pressure, HbA1c, and blood glucose than subjects in the Small Breakfast group. Body weight, body mass index, waist circumference, and hip circumference declined similarly in both groups. A significantly greater proportion of the subjects in the Big Breakfast group reduced their dose of diabetes medication, while a significantly greater proportion of those in the Small

Breakfast group *increased* their diabetes medication. The fat- and protein-rich Big Breakfast produced a feeling of satiety and reduced hunger in the participants. Thus, eating a high-fat, high-protein, low-carb breakfast might be a simple way to help manage or even prevent type 2 diabetes[81].

A study in Spain found that earlier consumption of the biggest meal of the day improved weight loss. Overweight and obese persons at weight-loss clinics in Spain participated in a program that featured the Mediterranean diet and behavioral- and cognitive-change techniques. Over 20 weeks, participants who ate lunch—the biggest meal of the day—before 3:00 p.m. lost significantly more weight (about 2.1 kg) than participants who ate lunch after 3:00 p.m. Surprisingly, both groups had similar energy intake, dietary composition, appetite hormones, sleep, and physical activity[82].

Americans typically eat about half of their daily protein at dinner. However, recent studies suggest that eating equal amounts of protein (25-30 grams) at breakfast, lunch, and dinner promotes greater skeletal muscle protein synthesis. Improving skeletal muscle strength can be especially important for older people to help prevent frailty[83].

Supplements

Supplements are highly controversial in the medical community. Claims about their effectiveness vary widely. A meta-analysis in the *Journal of the American Medical Association*[84] showed that supplementation with antioxidant vitamins, including beta-carotene, vitamin A, or vitamin E, may increase mortality. A large-scale, randomized trial found a daily multivitamin found a modest but statistically significant 8 percent reduces risk of cancer of 11 years of follow-up[85]. A 2013 editorial in *Annals of Internal Medicine* stated that "supplementing diet of well-nourished adults with (most) mineral or vitamin supplements has no clear benefit and might even be harmful." A 2018 article in the *Journal of the American Medical Association* stated that "most randomized clinical trials of vitamin and mineral supplements have not demonstrated clear benefits for primary or secondary prevention of chronic diseases not related to nutritional deficiency"[86]. In spite of the controversy, over half of Americans take at least one supplement.

Based on what I see people buying at my local grocery store, it's hard for me to believe that many of those people are well nourished with respect to vitamins and minerals. I rarely see shoppers loading their carts with fresh veggies and fruits. Rather, I see carts brimming with sodas, other sweetened drinks, chips, and other foods that don't appear on lists of healthful things to eat. The scientific literature supports the conclusion that at least some supplements probably support better health for some people. Recommendations for vitamins are based on preventing vitamin deficiencies, not providing an optimum level of health. Yes, supplements can cause problems. But, again, the scientific literature indicates that those problems can likely be avoided with a modicum of background research. Finally, blanket statements claiming that peer-reviewed studies do not support using supplements to improve health are misleading.

My overall conclusion with regard to supplements—vitamins, minerals, herbs/botanicals, or specialty supplements—is this: Do your homework before taking them. Make sure that any supplement you're considering has published research that backs up its safety and effectiveness. Make sure it doesn't create or exacerbate problems you already have. If you're taking medication, ask your doctor if the supplement might interact harmfully with your medication. Check out the company that markets a supplement regarding the firm's integrity, such as third-party testing.

Practical Ways to *Eat Better*

- **Pay more attention to how you feel before and after your eat.** Many people eat out of boredom or because they are stressed about something. A better approach is to eat when hungry and to stop eating when nearly full. In other words, eat more mindfully[87].

- **Pay more attention to what and how you eat.** I love ice cream. My love for it vastly exceeds my capacity to burn off the calories it contains. I hit upon a solution recently. If I discover ice cream in the freezer, I'll eat one tablespoon per day after dinner. I savor the flavor and remind myself that I'll burn off those calories during my after-dinner walk. I'll also remind myself that I'll feel better, be healthier, and be more able to continue my long-distance hiking and bicycling adventures (both are highly important to me) if I eat well—by enjoying ice cream in small amounts.

- **Leave ultraprocessed foods at the grocery store.** Avoid buying, or at least minimize, highly appealing yet highly ultraprocessed foods that contain lots of salt, sugar, unhealthy fats, calories, and additives so they don't constantly provide cues at home that promote you to overeat. A new study found that each 10 percent increase in ultraprocessed food consumption predicted a 14 percent higher risk of dying over a 7-year follow-up period[88].

- **Eat at home more often.** David Kessler's eye-opening book *The End of Overeating*[89] documents how the American food industry, including manufacturers and chain restaurants, developed precise combinations of fat, sugar, and salt, along with exotic flavorings that make foods hyperpalatable. Such foods have been designed to create intense sensory experiences, are readily available, and are easy to chew and swallow. Hyperpalatable foods are essentially irresistible, and prompt us to suspend rational judgement and eat indulgently[89].

- **Create an environment that helps you *Eat Better*.** We can make small changes in our environment to help us eat healthier. To help manage food consumption, buy food in small packages and keep the packages out of view when not in use. Serve food on or in small plates, bowls, and glasses. Leave serving bowls in the kitchen to minimize second helpings. Don't eat in front of the TV.

- **Eat intuitively.** Eating can be both satisfying and healthful. Tribole and Resch's book *Intuitive Eating* is geared toward veteran dieters. But its commonsense approach would likely help anyone *Eat Better*. Given the poor track record of dieting, I suggest you try eating intuitively to change your relationship with food.

Three Key Points

1. Ramp up consumption of colorful, non-starchy vegetables to at least five servings per day.

2. Minimize consumption of fruit juices, sweetened drinks, and ultraprocessed foods with added sugar or artificial sweeteners.

3. Shift food consumption to earlier in the day. Make breakfast or lunch the largest meal, and dinner the smallest.

Chapter 3

Sleep More and Better

Sleep has a critical role in promoting health.
—Michael R. Irwin[1]

One-third of Americans are sleep-deprived. According to the National Sleep Foundation (2008), Americans get two hours less sleep per night on average now than in 1960. For most people, habitually getting less than seven hours per night is associated with a variety of health problems, including increased risk of premature death, cardiovascular disease, immune system decline, obesity, type 2 diabetes, accidents, and some forms of cancer. Interestingly, long sleep duration is also associated with certain adverse outcomes. (More about that later.)

Poor sleep, a state of inadequate or mistimed sleep, arises from two sources: Primary sleep disorders and chronic sleep deficiency. The Institute of Medicine estimates that 50–70 million American adults have a sleep disorder. Such disorders include sleep apnea, insomnia, narcolepsy, and restless leg syndrome.

Sleep Problems

Obstructive sleep apnea and insomnia head the list of the most prevalent sleep problems. The former is often undiagnosed, yet it's a risk factor for several chronic diseases, such as obesity. Sleep problems can reflect both sleep duration and quality.

Obstructive sleep apnea

Obstructive sleep apnea is characterized by repeated collapse of the airway and reduced oxygen in the blood. It is the most common form of sleep apnea and contributes greatly to daytime drowsiness in seniors. About one-fourth of seniors have undiagnosed sleep apnea[2]. Scientists measure the severity of sleep apnea using the apnea-hypopnea index, or AHI, which represents the number of apnea or hypopnea events per hour.

To clarify the relationship between obstructive sleep apnea (OSA) and exercise capacity, researchers studied two groups of subjects: one with newly diagnosed but untreated moderate to severe OSA (more than 15 AHI events per hour), and a control group with mild or no OSA (fewer than 15 AHI events per hour). The AHI was significantly higher for the severe OSA subjects than the control subjects. The maximum rate of oxygen consumption was significantly lower in the moderate to severe OSA group compared to the control group, after controlling for potentially confounding variables. Impaired exercise capacity might be a mechanism that explains the observed relationship between fatal and nonfatal cardiovascular events and OSA[3].

Insomnia

Chronic insomnia is a major problem for primary care providers. Patients' sleep problems typically include difficulty falling asleep, difficulty maintaining sleep, early morning awakening, and non-restorative sleep. Previous research suggests that nurse-administered sleep counseling based on cognitive behavioral therapy (CBT) might be effective and cost-effective. Wait-listed patients served as the control group. Swedish and UK researchers designed a random-ized controlled trial to test the clinical effectiveness of a CBT program in an environment similar to a "real-world" primary care setting.

Nurses and social workers delivered the CBT-based program to participants recruited in five district health care centers in small Swedish cities and towns. By coincidence, all of the nurses and social workers had prior training in CBT. The nurses attended an additional two-day training as part of this study.

Cognitive behavioral therapy helps people recognize and challenge negative thoughts, beliefs, and behavior patterns about themselves and the larger world. The desired result is to develop more helpful thought patterns to cope effectively with life's challenges.

Just under half of the participants in the CBT group showed clinically meaningful improvements in sleep. Members of the CBT group significantly improved the main outcome, the Insomnia Severity Index, while those in the control group did not. Furthermore, members of the CBT group showed a clinically meaningful reduction in both time to fall asleep and wake time after sleep onset. However, the positive effects of the CBT intervention (developing more useful beliefs about themselves and the world) deteriorated rapidly after the study ended. While CBT improved sleep in the short term, it did not instill long-term positive sleep habits in the participants. This study highlights the need to turn healthy choices into healthy habits to maintain positive long-term changes[4].

Researchers suggest three ways to improve overall health through better sleep health: (1) recognize and regularly meet the biological requirement for sleep, (2) synchronize sleep with the body's natural daily biological rhythms, and (3) recognize the symptoms of sleep disorders and seek medical attention if symptoms appear[5].

Benefits Linked to *Sleep More and Better*

Does getting eight hours of restful sleep each night promote our health and well-being? Most of us would probably respond, "Yes!" But we may not appreciate the extent to which sufficient restful sleep promotes our health and well-being. Sleep duration and quality are both important. Consider the following list of benefits linked to getting plenty of regular, restful sleep.

Benefits Linked to
Sleep More and Better

- Greater longevity
- Bodily restoration and repair
- Waste products removed from brain
- Day's events solidified into permanent memory
- Improved motor skill memory
- Improved immune system function
- Diminished stress response

Greater longevity

Do elders have different sleep patterns than younger persons? If so, might those patterns affect longevity? To find out, Brazilian researchers used subjects from the Elderly Epidemiologic Study, plus additional volunteers recruited from São Paulo. Thirty-eight participants spent a night at a sleep laboratory. The "oldest old" (ages 85–105 years) showed lower sleep efficiency and lower rapid eye movement (REM) sleep—commonly known as the dreaming stage—than the older adults (60–70 years). The quantity and quality of slow-wave sleep (SWS)—the most restorative sleep stage—did not differ across the oldest old, older adult, and young adult (20–30 years) groups. The oldest old maintained more regular sleep-wake schedules than the older adults, and had more favorable blood lipid profiles (higher HDL cholesterol and lower triglycerides) than the other groups. The study showed that regular sleep patterns, maintenance of SWS, and a favorable lipid profile predicted greater longevity[6].

Other studies regarding the relationship between amounts of sleep and the risk of death and cardiovascular diseases show conflicting findings. The largest review and meta-analysis as of 2017 included 67 published articles and sought to determine the amount of sleep that predicted the lowest risk of all-cause mortality and cardiovascular events for generally healthy people. Sample sizes of studies ranged from 724 to 1,116,936 participants. The lowest risks of all-cause mortality, total cardiovascular events, coronary heart disease, and stroke were associated with approximately seven hours of sleep per night. Overall, the risk of these conditions rose more steeply with *increasing* daily sleep and dropped less steeply with *decreasing* daily sleep. For example, people getting six or eight hours of daily sleep had a six and 13 percent higher risk of dying prematurely, respectively, compared to those getting seven hours of daily sleep. This report contradicts part of the oft-repeated exhortation to get 7–9 hours of restful sleep per night. The authors suggest that longer sleep duration may reflect obstructive sleep apnea, depression, low-socioeconomic status, low household income, and low education—all possible markers of conditions that elevate mortality and cardiovascular risk. Thus, getting more than seven but less than nine hours of sleep may predict but not cause an increased risk in mortality and cardiovascular disease[7].

Another study followed 37 men and 72 women (average age 80 years) in the village of Ogimi in Okinawa, Japan, which has a high proportion of centenarians. Elderly persons who exhibited good sleep health took short naps, exercised regularly or walked, maintained regular eating habits, and ate lots of seaweed and fish over a 10-year period. The elderly with good sleep health also had higher participation in senior citizens clubs compared to those without good sleep health, indicating high emotional adaptability of the good sleepers. Unsurprisingly, healthy lifestyle choices predict better overall health among the elderly[8].

Bodily restoration and repair

Resting provides an opportunity for our body to repair itself. The restoration theory of sleep, developed by British researcher Ian Oswald and others, centers on the idea that sleep restores various biological functions. Different phases of the sleep cycle may promote different types of reorganization and repair. For example, rapid eye movement sleep is necessary for brain growth, repair, and reorganization. Slow-wave sleep (SWS) promotes bodily growth and repair. During SWS, growth hormone is released, which promotes protein synthesis that supports bodily restoration and repair. More recently, Horne expanded Oswald's theory. Horne suggested that sleep is divided into core sleep (including REM and SWS) and optional sleep. He suggested that both brain restoration and repair take place during core sleep. Bodily restoration occurs during optional sleep, as well other times, such as during periods of relaxed wakefulness.

Waste products removed from brain

Despite thousands of studies, science has yet to understand fully why sleep is restorative or why the lack of sleep impairs brain function. Recent research with mice sheds new light on these mysteries. The lymphatic system, which removes waste materials from most of our body, does not exist in the brain. Rather, cerebrospinal fluid that circulates between the neurons removes waste materials from our brain that build up during waking hours. Researchers in New York found that both natural sleep and anesthesia were associated with a 60 percent increase in the space between brain cells. This space helps the brain flush out toxins linked with neurodegenerative diseases. Thus, the clearance of metabolic waste during sleep may account, in part, for its restorative capability. While mice aren't humans, this research hints that waste products might be similarly removed from human brains[9].

Day's events solidified into permanent memory

During sleep, our brain solidifies the previous day's events into permanent memory. Additionally, sequences of learned skills become muscle memory during REM sleep[2].

While earlier research focused on the role of REM sleep on the brain, recent studies show the importance of slow-wave sleep for memory consolidation. The waking brain seems to optimize memory encoding, whereas the sleeping brain appears to optimize memory consolidation. During SWS, consolidation arises from reactivating recently encoded neuronal memories and transforming them for integration into long-term memory. Follow-up REM sleep may stabilize these transformed memories[10].

Improved motor skill memory

Sleep appears to improve motor skill learning. Researchers at Harvard investigated whether a period of sleep or a period of wakefulness following motor skill training would lead to greater improvement in a motor skill task. The task involved tapping the number keys on a computer keyboard with the nondominant left hand in the order 4-1-3-2-4. Sixty-two healthy young adults tapped this number sequence as quickly and as accurately as possible for 30 seconds, followed by 30 seconds of rest. This regimen was repeated 12 times. The greatest degree of improvement from test to retest occurred when sleep (averaging 7.6 hours) occurred between test and retest. Subjects in one group were monitored in a sleep laboratory. Subjects with the highest amount of non-REM sleep, especially late at night, showed the greatest improvement in finger tapping at retest. Thus, post-training sleep may be required for optimal consolidation of motor skill learning[11].

A follow-up study by these Harvard researchers confirmed significant increases in tapping-performance speed following one night of sleep, with modest additional increases in performance speed following three more nights of sleep. Motor skill learning seems to include two steps: the first depends on training, and the second depends on sleep. Getting enough restful sleep appears to be critical for learning new motor skills[12].

Improved immune system function

Both sleep and our daily biological (circadian) rhythms strongly affect immune system function. Sleep disturbances have a powerful influence on the risk of contracting an infectious disease, the incidence and progression of several chronic diseases, and the onset of depression. Even a single night of poor sleep stresses the body.

The immune system has two branches: innate and adaptive. Innate immunity, the body's first line of defense, refers to the proliferation of specific cells that respond with inflammatory responses to injuries and microbial pathogens. Adaptive immunity kicks into play when pathogens evade or overcome the innate immune defenses. Sleep loss impairs adaptive immunity, including responses to vaccines, and predicts inflammation. Prolonged poor sleep leads to increased markers of inflammatory activity. Chronic, low-level inflammation is associated with type 2 diabetes, cardiovascular disease, and other chronic conditions. Improving sleep and reducing stress may reduce both inflammation and the risk of cardiovascular disease[1].

A recent review concluded that adequate, regular, restful sleep helps establish immunological memory; that is, our body can respond more readily to pathogens when our immune system is primed to defend against attack by specific pathogens. Vaccination studies show that a single night of normal sleep following vaccination promotes better immune response to the vaccination. These positive effects persist for a year. On the flip side, immunological response declines after six days of restricted sleep[13].

Deep slow-wave sleep may also strengthen immunological memories of previously encountered pathogens. The immune system "remembers" bacteria and viruses by collecting pieces of the microbes to create memory T cells. Studies in humans show that long-term increases in memory T cells are associated with deep slow-wave sleep during nights after vaccination. Thus, slow-wave sleep may help form long-term body memories, which may lead to adaptive behavioral and immunological responses. It follows that sleep deprivation may put our body at higher risk for infection[14].

Diminished stress response

Sleep More and Better can increase our ability to adapt to life's stressors. Recent evidence suggests that poor sleep in adults affects the relationship between stressful events in life and the stress response, as measured by production of the stress hormone cortisol. Stressful events may not trigger a stress response in well-rested adults, but the same stressors might trigger a stress response in sleep-deprived adults. The same findings also apply to children and adolescents. In a study of 220 young people, ages 8–18, in Montreal, sleep quality and duration influenced the association between perceived stress, stressful events, and daily stress response, as measured by saliva cortisol levels. Sleep deprivation can diminish our ability to *Defuse Chronic Stress*[15] (see chapter 5). The study provides a compelling reason to *Sleep More and Better*.

Poor Outcomes Linked to Failing to *Sleep More and Better*

Inadequate sleep health is an underappreciated contributor to ill overall health. As noted above, sleep duration—primarily short as opposed to long—and sleep disorders are associated with numerous adverse health outcomes[16]. The risk of experiencing these bad outcomes increases from failing to *Sleep More and Better*.

Poor Outcomes Linked to Failing to *Sleep More and Better*	Premature death
	Cardiovascular disease
	Type 2 diabetes
	Obesity
	Dementia
	Hypertension
	Reduced self-control
	Poorer performance and attendance at work
	Diminished executive functions
	Diminished bone health
	Accidents
	Biological aging

Premature death

Would you believe that sleep patterns can influence our chances of dying prematurely? Researchers studied 185 healthy older adults, primarily in their 60s through 80s, with no history of mental illness, sleep complaints, or current cognitive impairment. The subjects were enrolled in one of eight research protocols between October 1981 and February 1997 that included assessments of electrical activity in the brain (using an EEG test) during sleep. During a follow-up period of roughly 13 years, 66 individuals died, 118 were still living, and the fate of one was uncertain. Individuals who took longer than 30 minutes to fall asleep had a two-fold greater risk of premature death than those who took less than 30 minutes to fall asleep. Older adults who took a long time to fall asleep had a higher risk of dying beyond that associated with age, gender, or medical burden. Interventions that improve older adults' sleep initiation, continuity, and quality may help them live longer[17].

Cardiovascular disease

Sleep apnea and milder types of sleep-disordered breathing are associated with cardiovascular stress. One cross-sectional study sought to determine if the association extended to cardiovascular disease. Subjects included 6,424 community-dwelling people who underwent one night of unsupervised monitoring of sleep variables. The odds of having at least one type of self-reported cardiovascular disease increased as the degree of the sleep apnea–hypopnea index (AHI) increased, from 1.00 in the lowest quartile (the reference group) to 1.42 in the highest quartile. Cardiovascular diseases occurred in AHI ranges (the number of apneas or hypopneas recorded per hour of sleep) considered normal or only a little abnormal (1–10 events per hour). Thus, even minor sleep disorders may increase the risk of cardiovascular disease[18].

Pooled data from 16 studies showed that *mild* obstructive sleep apnea was not associated with major adverse cardiac events, coronary heart disease, stroke, cardiac death, all-cause death, or heart failure. However, *moderate* obstructive sleep apnea predicted increased risk of coronary disease. *Severe* obstructive sleep apnea predicted major adverse cardiac events, coronary heart disease, stroke, cardiac death, or all-cause death, especially for men[19]. If you think you might have major sleep apnea, seek medical advice.

Research shows that long sleep duration is associated with increased risk of cardiovascular events. Could too much sleep create arterial problems? In a recent study, researchers examined the association between sleep duration and sleep quality in a large sample of young and middle-aged adults with no symptoms of arterial disease. Extreme sleep duration and poor subjective sleep quality were associated with increased prevalence of artery calcification and greater artery stiffness. The results highlight the importance of adequate—but not excessive—quantity and quality of sleep to maintain cardiovascular health[20].

Type 2 diabetes

Sleep deprivation can reduce blood glucose tolerance (which leads to excessive blood sugar levels) and increase insulin resistance (which predicts increased risk of type 2 diabetes). Thus, short sleep duration might promote type 2 diabetes. Researchers examined data from 8,992 subjects over 8–10 years in the first National Health and Nutrition Examination Survey (NHANES 1) to determine if short sleep duration might be risk factors for type 2 diabetes. Relative to subjects who reported seven hours of sleep per night, those who reported five or fewer had 47 percent higher risk of developing type 2 diabetes. If short sleep increases insulin resistance and decreases glucose tolerance, then improved sleep duration (up to a point) and better quality sleep may help prevent type 2 diabetes[21].

Australian researchers analyzed data from the 45 and Up Study, a long-term study of 191,728 or 156,902 subjects, depending on the statistical models used. The researchers found a significant association between less than six hours of sleep per night and a risk of type 2 diabetes. Furthermore, a meta-analysis of 10 other published studies showed a significant association between short sleep and diabetes risk. Short sleep was associated with about a 30 percent higher risk of developing type 2 diabetes compared to subjects who got seven hours of sleep per night[22].

Obesity

People who regularly sleep 7 or fewer hours per night are more likely to have a high body mass index and be obese than people who get more sleep, according to a recent review of published studies. Sleep reduction is associated with increased levels of the hormone ghrelin and markers of inflammation. Ghrelin promotes appetite and is secreted by the stomach when it's empty. Sleep reduction is also associated with lower levels of the hormone leptin (secreted by fat cells, it suppresses appetite) and insulin sensitivity[23].

The hormones leptin and ghrelin help regulate how much we eat. A study involving 12 healthy men investigated how daytime concentrations of these hormones varied after two consecutive nights of sleep deprivation (four hours per night) or sleep extension (10 hours per night). Compared to subjects with four hours of sleep, those with 10 hours of sleep exhibited lower leptin (less appetite suppression) and higher ghrelin (greater appetite promotion) levels. Hunger and appetite ratings increased more in subjects with four hours of sleep compared to those with 10 hours of sleep. Thus, changes in levels of leptin and ghrelin following sleep deprivation would favor increased food consumption[24]. Hormonal imbalance could account for the observation that losing weight is difficult for sleep-deprived or long-sleeping people[25].

Accumulating research suggests that sleep deprivation, either from behavior or disease, promotes obesity. In the 2008 "Sleep in America" report, American adults reported that they need an average of seven hours and 18 minutes of sleep per night to function well. Yet 44 percent of respondents got less than seven hours of sleep per night. Sixteen percent got less than six hours on a typical weeknight. Research shows that people who sleep six hours per night have a 23 percent higher chance of being obese; with five hours per night, the risk rises to 50 percent[2]. Sleep-deprivation may interact with the American obesogenic food environment to promote overeating and weight gain. Limited sleep may also lead to lethargy with lower amounts of physical activity[26].

Interestingly, the rise in obesity in developed countries parallels the rise in obstructive sleep apnea. Obstructive sleep apnea affects about 14 percent of Americans. The connection between insufficient sleep and obesity may be mediated through the hormones leptin and ghrelin. Leptin levels rise with higher amounts of sleep, while ghrelin levels decline. The opposite occurs in sleep-deprived persons. Furthermore, research shows that both sleep deprivation and poor sleep quality interfere with glucose metabolism, reducing glucose tolerance and insulin sensitivity. Thus, increased appetite caused by a decrease in leptin and an increase in ghrelin (with attendant weight gain) coupled with problematic glucose metabolism (poor blood sugar control) could account for increased risk of obesity for persons who get insufficient and/or low-quality sleep[27].

Dementia

Sleep disturbances appear to increase the risk of cognitive impairment, but a newly published review and meta-analysis of longitudinal studies found that they also increase the risk of Alzheimer's disease and other dementias. The 18 studies included 246,786 subjects. When different types of sleep disturbances—insomnia, sleep-disordered breathing, and others—were combined, individuals with one or more sleep disturbances had significant 19, 49, and 47 percent higher risks of all-cause dementia, Alzheimer's disease, and vascular dementia, respectively, compared to individuals without sleep disturbance. Vascular dementia refers to cognitive problems caused by inadequate blood flow to the brain. Individuals with sleep-disordered breathing had 18 and 20 percent higher risks of all-cause dementia and Alzheimer's disease, respectively, compared to individuals without such disturbances. Among different types of sleep disturbances, only sleep-disordered breathing was significantly related to risk of vascular dementia[28].

Hypertension

Growing evidence suggests that insufficient restful sleep predicts hypertension. Chinese researchers conducted a meta-analysis of 11 prospective studies of habitual sleep duration or symptoms of insomnia in relation to hypertension. Short sleep duration, sleep continuity disturbance, early morning awakening, and combined symptoms of insomnia predicted significantly increased risk of hypertension[29].

The relationship between sleep duration and hypertension is stronger for females than males and stronger for middle-aged people than younger or elderly persons. One study showed that increasing daily sleep duration by 35 minutes reduced systolic and diastolic blood pressure by 14 and 8 mm Hg, respectively, both of which are clinically significant. If we *Sleep More and Better*, we may reduce our risk of hypertension[30].

Reduced self-control

Sleep deprivation appears to reduce self-control. Being able to control our impulses is key to successfully avoiding or overcoming unhealthy temptations. It's useful to think of three aspects of self-control: (1) things we want to do or do more of, (2) things we do not want to do or want to do less of, and (3) long-term goals where we want to focus our energy. Lack of sleep impairs our body's metabolism of glucose, the brain's main source of energy. Our brain is our body's greatest user of glucose on a per-pound basis. A shortage of glucose increases our desire for sweets and caffeine. Glucose insufficiency hampers the operation of our prefrontal cortex, the seat of self-control. Happily, the effects of short-term sleep deprivation appear to be reversible with a good night's snooze[31].

Self-awareness is the bedrock of self-control. Being distracted (for example, trying to do two things at once) reduces self-awareness and, therefore, self-control. Most of us have competing desires: We want to eat a donut, but we also want to avoid junk food. We also make choices on autopilot without conscious self-awareness of what's driving those choices, or of their long-term consequences in our lives. Looking from the positive side, we can improve our self-awareness with focused attention, meditation, and mindfulness. If we develop a habit of being aware of temptations and making healthy choices, we'll be miles ahead in the long run. Change is often difficult. To make change easier, start with small steps[31] to *Sleep More and Better.*

Poorer performance and attendance at work

Sleep deprivation leads to poorer health and poorer performance at work[2,32]. A new study investigated the relationship between sleep habits and employee productivity among 598,676 participants in employer-sponsored health and wellness programs in a variety of industries. Researchers gathered information on employees' self-reported hours of sleep, fatigue, absence days, and presenteeism (working while sick). The least productivity loss occurred among employees who reported eight hours of sleep at night. More daytime fatigue predicted more absence and more presenteeism. Companies that offer health and wellness programs may realize greater value and greater productivity by promoting better sleep habits of their employees[33].

Researchers investigated the effects of sleep disturbances on 4,188 randomly selected employees at four U.S. corporations. The employees were classified in one of four groups: insomnia, insufficient sleep syndrome, at-risk, or good sleep. On average, these subjects reported needing 7.6 hours of sleep per day to feel rested but reported getting only 6.4 hours. In general, sleep disturbances were associated with lower work productivity, impaired work performance, and poorer safety outcomes. Compared to the at-risk and good sleep groups, participants in the insomnia and insufficient sleep syndrome groups reported significantly greater time as "performance limited" in terms of time management, mental/interpersonal demands, output demands, and physical job demands. Work productivity loss increased from 2.5 percent in the good sleep group to 6.5 percent in the insomnia group. Similarly, the insomnia and insufficient sleep syndrome groups showed greater impairment in job performance criteria of attention, decision making, memory, and motivation. Safety outcomes, such as unintentional sleep at work, injuries at home due to sleepiness, nodding off while driving, and near-miss or actual accidents due to sleepiness were all greater for the insomnia and insufficient sleep syndrome groups compared to the at-risk and good sleep groups. Moreover, the annual per capita economic cost of poor sleep, primarily borne by employers, ranged from $1,293 for the good sleep group to $3,156 for the insomnia group[34].

In a sample of Finnish adults, sleep disturbances—including insomnia-related symptoms, early morning awakening, being more tired than others, and using sleeping pills—each significantly predicted a greater absence from work due to sickness. The amounts of sleep associated with the lowest risk of sleep absence were 7.6 and 7.8 hours for women and men, respectively. Researchers estimated that eliminating sleep disturbances would reduce direct costs of absence from work due to sickness by 28 percent[35]. Another Finnish study of 10 years duration recruited City of Helsinki employees as subjects. After controlling for smoking, alcohol use, physical activity, and fruit/vegetable intake, *poor sleep quality alone* predicted higher costs to the city due to employee sickness, compared to employees with good sleep quality[36].

Diminished executive functions

Insufficient sleep precipitates a host of undesirable mental outcomes, including reduced alertness, attention, and concentration, as well as diminished executive functions, such as problem solving, impulse control, and decision making. Studies have shown that the function of the brain's prefrontal cortex is especially sensitive to sleep deprivation. Dysfunction in the prefrontal cortex is associated with impaired emotional intelligence and poor constructive thinking.

Researchers at the Walter Reed Army Hospital in Maryland recruited 26 healthy military volunteers to test the hypothesis that sleep deprivation would lead to both impaired emotional intelligence and impaired constructive thinking in a controlled laboratory setting. Fifty-five hours of sleep deprivation produced statistically significant declines in overall emotional intelligence and specifically in stress management, intra- and intrapersonal functioning. With respect to constructive thinking, the subjects showed reduced behavioral coping and increased esoteric thinking. This study supports previous research suggesting that sleep deprivation impairs prefrontal cortex activity, which leads to temporary disruption of executive functions[37].

Older people typically exhibit declines in aspects of cognitive performance; one possible explanation is declining sleep quality and/or quantity, which is also typical of older people. Researchers used data from 157 volunteers aged 65–80 years who were recruited for an aging study. The subjects did not necessarily exhibit sleep problems. Each volunteer completed a number of tests designed to measure aspects of cognitive performance. The good sleepers exhibited significantly lower (more healthful) scores on the Geriatric Depression Scale, a "yes/no" screening tool used to measure depression in older adults. Moreover, good sleepers exhibited significantly higher (more healthful) scores for tests that assessed cognitive performance in working memory, attention shifting, and abstract reasoning. Good and poor sleepers did not differ in information-processing speed, inhibitory function, verbal memory, or mood. Thus, poor sleep may diminish certain, but not all, aspects of cognitive performance[38].

Diminished bone health

Researchers in Oregon investigated the relationship between sleep, bone disorders, and fractures. Their findings indicated that obstructive sleep apnea can adversely affect bone strength and the formation of new bone tissue via several pathways. A future concern is the increasing prevalence of childhood obesity, which increases the risk of obstructive sleep apnea and, potentially, damage to developing bones[39].

In 2010, about 54 million American adults over age 50 were affected by low bone mass. Ten million of those were in the range of osteoporosis. In 2005, osteoporotic fractures cost Americans an estimated $19 billion. These fractures are associated with several undesirable outcomes, including reduced quality of life, higher risk of institutionalization, and increased risk of dying (from hip fractures). A recent review of the scientific literature concluded that sleep apnea impairs bone health and increases the risk of osteoporosis and factures[39].

Accidents

A substantial fraction of traffic accidents worldwide arises from insufficient and/or disordered sleep. Research shows that driver fatigue accounts for 16–20 percent of major highway accidents in the UK, Australia, and Brazil. Fatigue can develop from sleep disorders, especially obstructive sleep apnea, excessive workload, and lack of physical and mental rest. Greater awareness of the importance of sleep may help reduce the frequency of sleep-related accidents[40].

Strategies to reduce the frequency of sleep-related accidents include:

1. Educational programs to raise awareness that short or disordered sleep can cause traffic accidents

2. Physical exercise to increase alertness and promote better sleep

3. Substances, like caffeine, that promote alertness

4. Educational programs that promote treatment of sleep disorders

5. Use of continuous positive airway pressure (CPAP) devices to help reduce sleepiness among drivers with obstructive sleep apnea

Biological aging

A 2015 study by researchers at UCLA suggested that a single night of partial sleep deprivation promotes biological aging in older adults. One night of partial sleep deprivation was shown to activate gene expression patterns in a type of cell (peripheral blood mononuclear cells) that reduced the cells' inability to perform necessary functions. Functional limitations increased the cells' susceptibility to senescence, a process thought to contribute to aging. The UCLA study supports the hypothesis that sleep deprivation is associated with elevated disease risk because it promotes molecular processes involved in biological aging[41].

A follow-up study by the UCLA group used DNA methylation, a process correlated to the epigenetic, or chronological, aging of cell types, to estimate the biological age of blood plasma cells in relation to insomnia and sleep duration. Study subjects included 2,078 participants (mean age 64) in the Women's Health Initiative. Symptoms of insomnia were associated with a measure of age acceleration, which suggests an aged immune system[42].

How Much Sleep is Enough?

Like much in science and medicine, there is no one-size-fits-all approach for how much sleep is enough or even ideal. For most of us, the amount of sleep we need tonight to perform optimally tomorrow probably lies between seven and eight hours per night. Some research shows that 9.25 hours of sleep per night are required, on average, for full alertness the next day[2], yet other studies suggest that this duration increases our risk of death and cardiovascular disease. We need to find out for ourselves the appropriate number of hours for us (see the following chart).

Nightly Sleep Durations

The National Sleep Foundation[43] convened an 18-member expert panel, representing 12 stakeholder organizations, to evaluate the scientific literature concerning sleep duration recommendations. The following guidelines recommended the duration of nightly sleep for healthy people with normal sleep (not suffering from a sleep disorder). Sleep durations outside the recommended range may be appropriate, but deviating far from the range is not recommended.

Age Group	Recommended Hours of Sleep
Newborns	14-17
Infants	12-15
Toddlers	11-14
Preschoolers	10-13
School-aged children	9-11
Teenagers	8-10
Young adults	7-9
Older adults	7-8

Seniors with four or more medical conditions are more likely to sleep less than six hours per night and experience daytime drowsiness than those with no medical conditions. Adults with positive moods/ outlooks and actively engaged lifestyles are more likely to sleep 7–9 hours per night and experience fewer nighttime complaints[2].

Practical Ways to *Sleep More and Better*

- **Create an ideal sleep environment.** You'll enjoy more restful sleep if your bedroom has these elements: (1) a comfortable bed, which mostly results from a high-quality mattress, (2) a comfortable pillow, (3) cool room air temperature, (4) moderate relative humidity, (5) darkness, and (6) quiet. In addition, I recommend keeping the TV out of the bedroom to reduce the temptation to watch late-night programs.

- **Find your ideal sleep duration.** To help you determine what length of nightly sleep works best for you, try this: For two weeks, keep a pad of paper next to your bed. Note the time you turn out the lights each night, the time you wake up and how you feel the next morning. Over the course of two weeks, you'll discover your optimal length of nightly sleep. I did this and found that I need 8.5 hours of sleep per night to wake up refreshed.

- **Develop a regular sleep schedule.** Research shows that going to bed and getting up at the same time every morning promotes better sleep. Once we know how many hours of sleep we need each night, we can set a target time for lights out in the evening and awakening in the morning.

- **Write expressively.** Patients with insomnia frequently report that they are unable to fall asleep due to unwanted thoughts and worries. Mind chatter can arise from the incomplete processing of daytime stressors and hassles. Expressive writing is a technique developed by James Pennebaker and Sandy Beall at the University of Texas in 1986. Writing about worries and concerns, with an emphasis on expressing and processing emotions, has been shown to reduce the time of sleep onset for poor sleepers. It can also diminish the effects of certain stressors and facilitate emotional processing[44]. Consider writing for a short period of time, say, 15 minutes, about a significant or even traumatic life event in a way that expresses your deepest feelings and emotions. Choose a time during the day when you can write without being interrupted. Expressing, evaluating, and synthesizing your thoughts and feelings about a highly personal topic in writing may improve your sleep[45].

- **Take short naps.** Older people often have trouble sleeping. A study in Japan showed that short (20 minute) naps after lunch and exercise at moderate intensity in the evening helped seniors awaken more quickly after sleep onset and improve sleep efficiency. Thus, sleep quality improved. At the end of the study, the mental health, volition, and physical health of the subjects also improved[46].

- **Turn off screens (TV, computer, cell phone) at least 30 minutes prior to bedtime.** The proliferation of devices with screens means that most of us are exposed to artificial light at night. Short wavelength light (typical of screens) significantly disrupts sleep continuity and organization. Short wavelength (bluish) light also leads to greater self-reported sleepiness and reduced attention the following morning. Exposure to several hours of artificial light from screens before bed time may reduce sleep quality and its restorative effects[47].

- **After preparing for bed, listen to a guided meditation, then go to sleep.** Just before going to bed, I often listen to a 12-minute guided meditation I found on the internet. I usually sit in my comfy office chair with the meditation playing on my laptop and cover the screen to block its light. The meditation helps me relax and fall asleep more quickly.

Three Key Points

1. Insufficient quantity and quality of sleep predict a host of health and work performance problems.

2. Going to bed and walking up at the same time every day will help you get enough sleep on a regular basis.

3. Creating an ideal sleep environment in your bedroom will help you get quality sleep on a regular basis.

Part 2

Nurture Your Mind with Three Healthy Choices

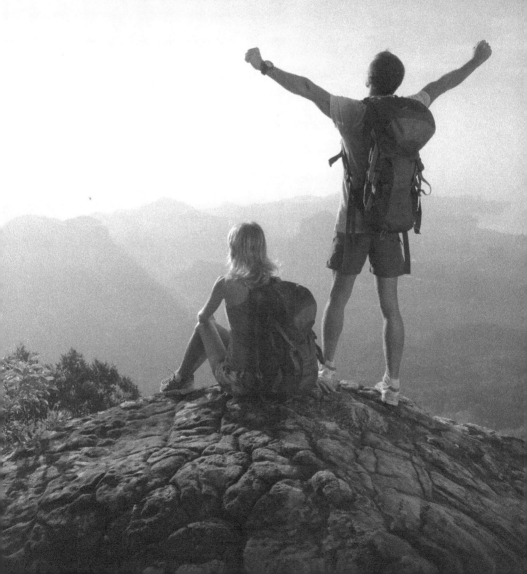

Chapter 4

Cultivate Social Connections

Throughout our lives, we are shaped and enriched
by the supportive surround of our relationships.
—George Vaillant[1]

Although many people consider physical exercise—including everyday activities such as washing dishes or doing the laundry—the most important thing we can do to create lifelong health and well-being, not everyone agrees. Leo Cooney, MD, who helped build the geriatrics program at the Yale School of Medicine, is quoted in the best-selling book *The Art of Aging* as saying, "Exercise is not the Holy Grail. If there's a Holy Grail, it's relationships with other people. In fact, if you have to decide between going to the gym and being with your grandchildren, I'd choose the grandchildren."

And consider this: In 1921, Lewis Terman of Stanford University recruited 1,500 young, bright children to determine whether he could predict the leaders of tomorrow as early as age 10. In summarizing the 80 years of follow-up research on the Terman group, authors Howard Friedman and Leslie Marin conclude in their book, *The Longevity Project*, that "social relations should be the first place to look for improving health and longevity."

In studies of centenarians around the world, Dan Buettner showed that only one lifestyle factor was common to all cultures with unusually high proportions of 100-year-olds: strong social connections[2]. The

MacArthur Foundation Study of Successful Aging found that social support leads not only to longer life but also to lower risk of arthritis, tuberculosis, depression, alcoholism, and decreases recovery time following surgery[3]. Karl Pillemer and his colleagues interviewed more than 1,000 older Americans about what made their lives worth living. He summarized the advice he heard most consistently in his inspiring book *30 Lessons for Living*. One of the lessons, "Emotional intelligence trumps every other kind," reminds us that if we *Cultivate Social Connections*, we'll recognize the primacy of connecting with others. Ideally, the interpersonal skills that we develop through our social connections—such as getting along with other people, learning from them, and serving them—will help us flourish.

John Rowe and Robert Kahn, in their influential book, *Successful Aging*, identified the main components of successful aging as: (1) absence of disease and disability and their predisposing factors, (2) maintenance of physical and cognitive function, and (3) continued involvement in social and productive pursuits.

Benefits Linked to *Cultivate Social Connections*

We humans are social animals. Our evolutionary history programmed us to be social to increase our likelihood of surviving accidents, injuries, and illness. Support may be a key benefit of a social network. Support comes in two flavors: instrumental and social. Instrumental refers to practical matters, such as getting a neighbor to help us replace the old sink in our bathroom. Social refers to emotional help, as in receiving consolation when our big project at work flops. In addition, support moves in several directions: from us to other people and from other people to us. Notably, *giving* support to others may be even more important than getting it.

Benefits Linked to
Cultivate Social Connections
- Greater quality of lifespan
- Increased longevity
- Improved cardiovascular health
- Increased happiness
- Better mental health
- Improved overall health and well-being
- Increased use of preventive services
- Better functional health
- Increased resistance to infection
- Reduced stress
- Greater cognitive function in old age
- Greater likelihood of post-traumatic growth

Greater quality of lifespan

Roseto is a small town in eastern Pennsylvania, founded primarily by people of Italian descent. During the town's early years, the men worked in nearby slate mines. In 1961, Doctors Stewart Wolf and John Bruhn met a local doctor, Benjamin Falcone, who remarked that the residents of Roseto experienced far lower rates of heart attacks than those of Bangor, a nearby town, where Dr. Falcone also practiced medicine. Wolf's and Bruhn's curiosity prompted them to study mortality records for 1955–1961. They learned that people in Roseto had half the death rate from coronary heart disease and from all causes compared to residents of nearby towns. The lower death rate occurred in spite of the prevalence of conventional risk factors for heart disease, including smoking, high cholesterol, and high-fat diets.

Interviews with residents of Roseto and research about relevant characteristics of the town led the doctors to hypothesize that the low death rate from coronary heart disease in Roseto arose from the strong community morale and the commitment of the residents to family and tradition. The way we perceive ourselves and others in our community apparently influences our health and well-being and that of our neighbors. Community solidarity and pride demand work, personal sacrifice, and concern for others.

Follow-up studies of the residents of Roseto revealed that the town's subsequent "Americanization" negated the health and well-being benefits of the previously close-knit community. Residents of Roseto shifted from holding family-centered values to self-centered, materialistic values. Comparison of death records for the 50-year period between 1935 and 1985 showed that after 1965, the mortality rate from heart attacks in Roseto caught up with that of Bangor[4].

Today, many of us work longer hours or are otherwise so preoccupied that we don't give social relationships the time and attention they deserve and require. Yet back in the fifties and sixties, the residents of Roseto created an emotionally supportive environment that, in turn, led to a much lower risk of heart disease[5].

Quality of Lifespan refers to length of life and the quality of that life. A higher quality of lifespan means living longer and better.

Increased Longevity

A 1988 article in *Science* summarized compelling early evidence from five studies showing that the link between social connections and mortality rivaled that of established health risk factors, such as smoking and high blood pressure[6].

In 2010, a group of researchers addressed this same connection. But instead of reviewing the five published studies from the *Science* article, they reviewed 148 studies. The larger group of studies showed overwhelmingly that a lack of social support is associated with mortality; 141 of the studies revealed a negative association (that is, as social relationships increased, mortality declined), while only seven revealed a positive association. Overall, the studies showed a 42 percent increase in the odds of survival for people with strong social relationships[7].

Two leading researchers recently concluded that "decades of research have documented an unequivocal influence of social connections on longevity"[8]. People who exhibited a high degree of social integration had a 91 percent increase in their odds of survival compared to people who had a low degree of social integration[7]. Therefore, interventions to improve social connections of older people could provide a major opportunity to increase longevity and *Quality of Lifespan.*

But what about the benefit of giving rather than receiving social support? Researchers at the University of Michigan investigated this question using data from the Changing Lives of Older Couples study. Subjects were drawn from a sample of 1,532 married couples in the Detroit metropolitan area. The husband of each couple was at least 65 years old when the study began. Individuals were followed until death or for five years (whichever happened first). Subjects who gave instrumental support to friends, neighbors, and relatives, and subjects who gave emotional support to their spouses both had a lower risk of mortality over the follow-up period. However, receiving support was not associated with reduced mortality when giving support was taken into account[9].

Research supports the somewhat counterintuitive idea that the benefit of social support accrues more to the giver than the receiver.

Japan exemplifies a high degree of social cohesion. One study investigated the link between social cohesion and mortality in 11,092 elderly people (aged 65–84 years) over a 10-year period in Japan's Shizuoka Prefecture. Social cohesion was evaluated from answers to four questions: (1) Do you get along with the people around you? (2) Are you satisfied with your friendships? (3) Do you have someone you can ask for a favor? (4) Are you satisfied with your relationships with the people around you? The sum of "yes" responses yielded a social cohesion score ranging from zero to four. A community cohesion score was obtained by summing the individual cohesion scores across 74 districts within the Shizuoka Prefecture. Higher *individual-level cohesion* was associated with lower all-cause mortality, cardiovascular mortality, pulmonary mortality, but not cancer mortality. However, no association appeared for *community-level cohesion* with any type of mortality. Thus, among older Japanese people, the longevity benefit of perceived high individual-level social cohesion did not translate into a longevity benefit for the larger community[10].

Improved cardiovascular health

In a report using data from 5,276 participants in the Health and Retirement Study (a nationally representative sample of older Americans), researchers found that perceived neighborhood social cohesion significantly predicted a reduced risk of heart attack. In 2006, a random sample of study participants completed a questionnaire that included four items relating to neighborhood social cohesion. Four years later, each standard deviation of increased perceived neighborhood social cohesion was associated with a 22 percent decline in risk of heart attack[11].

Better social connections could improve cardiovascular health via four pathways: (1) better lifestyle choices (greater physical activity, better nutrition, less smoking), (2) better physiological effects (lower stress, greater meaning in life, resourceful reappraisal of life events), (3) better medical adherence and compliance (taking medications according to prescription, following recommendations for diet and movement), and (4) improved biomarkers (reduced inflammation, blood pressure, blood fats)[8].

Increased happiness

While the vast majority of people want to be happy, psychologists seldom investigated happy people until the 21st Century. In 2002, two of the giants of the positive psychology movement, Ed Diener and Martin Seligman, produced an early, pivotal happiness study. Diener collected data from 222 undergraduates during a psychology course at the University of Illinois. Based on self-reports regarding the students' overall mood balance, daily mood balance, and life satisfaction, plus informant reports, the students were classified into three groups: (1) very happy (highest 10 percent), (2) average (middle 27 percent), and (3) very unhappy (lowest 10 percent). Members of the very happy group differed from both the average and very unhappy groups in terms of various measures, but none of the differences were statistically significant. The data showed that good social relationships were necessary but, by themselves, insufficient to be very happy. Not surprisingly, all 22 students in the very happy group had excellent social relationships. The very happy students experienced unpleasant emotions but were able subsequently to regain their emotional balance[12].

Better mental health

The Harvard Grant Study of Adult Development is a notable exception to the typical longitudinal study that follows groups of subjects for less than a decade. This unusual study began in 1939 when a group of Harvard sophomore men was selected for the study; additional sophomores were selected through 1944, for a total of 268 men. Over the ensuing decades, a mountain of data accumulated on these research participants.

George Vaillant's book *Triumphs of Experience* chronicles the lessons that he and other researchers gleaned from the first 75 years of this continuing study. Of the many lessons learned, Vaillant believes that the positive effect of an affectionate childhood rises to the top. Vaillant classified the Harvard men who ranked in the top quartile of a warm and supportive home environment as "cherished," while he classified those in the bottom quartile as "loveless." In their seventh decade of life, the loveless were eight times (!) more likely than the cherished to have experienced depression. This long-term study complements the findings of shorter-term studies that demonstrate the salutary effects of social support during adulthood[1].

Improved overall health and well-being

Social connections can reduce the incidence of such maladies as heart disease, cancer, and infectious diseases via two possible pathways: better health behaviors; and psychological processes linked to appraisals, emotions, moods, or feelings of control. Better health behaviors could include increasing exercise, improving diet, or not smoking. The psychological process of reappraisal could help defuse stressful situations[13].

Researchers in Louisiana used data from 771 participants in the Louisiana Healthy Aging Study to evaluate associations between social and physical activities with health across an age span from 21 to 101 years. Specifically, would the relationship between social activities and health previously observed by the research team still be present, even after controlling for levels of physical activity? Physical activity—measured as the number of hours spent outside the home—and social support both significantly predicted better self-reported health after controlling for sociodemographic factors. The number of clubs to which the subjects belonged significantly predicted objective health after controlling for sociodemographic factors. Further analysis revealed that social factors, even after accounting for physical activity, predicted better physical health. Thus, a network of social connections appears to help maintain good health into old age[14].

Dutch researchers conducted a longitudinal study to investigate a link between social connections and health. Using data from the Doetinchem Cohort Study in the Netherlands, the researchers asked whether positive or negative social experiences were associated with current or future health. At baseline, the researchers found that poor self-perceived overall health and poor self-perceived mental health were most prevalent in people with low levels of positive social experiences and with high levels of negative social experiences. After 10 years of follow-up, the odds of continued and/or newly developed poor mental health of participants with the lowest one-third of positive social experiences were 274 and 186 percent higher, respectively, than for those with the highest one-third of positive social experience. The odds of continued and/or newly developed poor mental health for people with the highest one-third of negative experiences of social support were 328 and 160 percent greater, respectively, than for the lowest one-third of negative experiences. Negative experiences of social support were associated with current smoking, physical inactivity, being overweight, and poor self-perceived health. Positive and negative experiences of social support are not simply opposites of each other; they independently predict better overall health[15].

It's widely known that people who own a pet can experience health benefits either due to the social support that a pet provides and/or from increased physical activity from having a pet, especially a dog. One recent review concluded that dog owners are likely to engage in more physical activity—mainly through dog walking—than people who don't own dogs. Evidence also indicates that the companionship of pets can reduce stress and bolster positive emotional states, leading to reduced autonomic nervous system activity, better cardiovascular function, and lower blood pressure[18].

An Australian study showed that health benefits from having a pet could also arise due to pets catalyzing social connections with neighbors. A telephone survey of 2,692 adult residents of Australia, California, Oregon, and Tennessee revealed that pet ownership predicted increased incidental social interactions and friendship formation with neighbors. The combination of increased social interactions and friendship formation further predicted increased informational, emotional, instrumental, and appraisal forms of social

Social Connections Promote Health Throughout Life

A recent study used data from four longitudinal studies to evaluate how social relationships affect overall health through various life stages. Social integration predicted better physiological function and lower risks of physical disorders across different life stages. The index of social integration included marital status; degree of contact with parents, children, and neighbors; and volunteering.

Outcomes varied among the different life stages. For example, social integration predicted a lower risk of inflammation and obesity in both adolescence and in late adulthood, but not in young adulthood or in young to mid-adulthood. Measures of perceived social support and strain predicted physiological markers differently than did social integration for mid-adulthood. Social integration appeared to be especially important during adolescence. Social deficits that occur during adolescence may lie dormant during young and middle adulthood, only to manifest support. Overall, 42 percent of pet owners reported receiving at least one of the foregoing forms of social support from people they met through their pet(s). Across the four geographical locations, pet owners were 61 percent more likely than non-pet owners to get to know neighbors they previously didn't know[19].

Pets can serve as a bridge between people who don't know each other. In addition, owning a pet can also help counter social isolation and loneliness, both of which are risk factors for poor health. Pets can help fulfill social connectivity needs, improve well-being, and provide an additional layer of social support on top of that provided by humans[20]. The positive health effects of dog ownership may be more pronounced for people living alone because they walk their dogs more and/or experience more social support than people living with others[21]. Fourteen years of walking our dog, Amelia, around our neighborhood connected my wife and me to people in our neighborhood far more than we anticipated.

during late adulthood. That said, the research showed that maintaining social connections is vital for a healthy late adulthood. The perceived quality of social relationships, rather than the density of social networks, may be a better measure of the benefit of social connections during adulthood. Social integration seems to promote better health and increase longevity across the life course[16].

The need to belong is a powerful, fundamental, and extremely pervasive motivator for humans to experience well-being[17].

Increased use of preventive services

Over the next decade, older Americans will account for half of the U.S. population. Given the projected doubling of the cost of U.S.

medical care by 2050 and the current underuse of preventive services by older people, improving the health of senior Americans appears to have a huge upside.

Several neighborhood characteristics have been shown to impact the use of preventive health services. Harvard researchers used data from 7,168 participants in the Health and Retirement Survey to determine if older people (average age of 69) in neighborhoods with better social cohesion would make greater use of preventive health services. The researchers found that higher perceived neighborhood social cohesion was significantly associated with greater use of flu vaccinations, cholesterol tests, mammograms, and pap smears, but not prostate screenings. (Lack of association with prostate screening might reflect that screenings cannot identify aggressive versus non-aggressive prostate cancer. Plus, diagnosing and treating prostate cancer entails considerable risks, including incontinence and impotence.) Consequently, neighborhood groups might be effective means to disseminate health information and increase its use by community elders[22].

Better functional health

The ability to perform all of one's activities of daily living greatly affects quality of life among older adults. Aspects of a woman's social network are significantly correlated with her functional status, regardless of other factors, according to a review of data for 56,436 U.S. women aged 55–72 enrolled in the Nurses' Health Study. Health and social network characteristics relative to healthy aging included physical functioning, role limitations, freedom from bodily pain, and vitality. Individual health risks, defined as current smoking, alcohol consumption, sedentary behavior, and being overweight, each contributed to significant reductions in functioning across all age groups. Having close friends, relatives, and a confidant strongly predicted high functioning among older women. On the flip side, absence of a confidant predicted reduced physical functioning and vitality. These negative effects were comparable in magnitude to those observed among women in the highest categories of smoking and body mass index[23].

A recent longitudinal study of Japanese persons investigated the effects of ties with family or relatives (either co-residing or living apart) upon functional health. The Japanese researchers used data from a study that followed 14,088 community-dwelling people age 65 or older at baseline. Compared to men who did not co-reside with family or receive support from friends or neighbors, men either co-residing with family or receiving support from friends and neighbors had a 19 and 15 percent lower risk, respectively, of becoming disabled over the 10-year follow-up period. This beneficial effect was not found for women, perhaps because they received lots of support regardless of their living situation[24]. The value provided from the support of friends and neighbors in reducing the risk of disability for men highlights the importance of *Cultivate Social Connections.*

Social Support Fosters Leisure Time Physical Activity

European researchers wanted to know if social support, either in the form of confiding/emotional or practical (such as help with moving about) from a close person, would predict a greater likelihood of getting the recommended amount of leisure time physical activity. The researchers used data from civil service office workers aged 35–55 at 20 government departments in London as part of the Whitehall II study. Workers who reported high social support of the confiding/emotional variety for the previous 12 months were more likely to report getting the recommended level of leisure time physical activity during the follow-up period, compared to people with little or none of this type of social support. Similarly, high practical support was associated with maintaining or improving recommended levels of leisure time physical activity during five years of follow-up. Practical support also predicted a generally more active lifestyle[25].

Increased resistance to infection

A diverse network of friends and family can increase resistance to infection by the common cold. Two hundred seventy-six healthy subjects from the Pittsburgh, Pennsylvania, area were quarantined then given nasal drops with one of two types of rhinovirus, which causes the common cold. The rate of infection declined as the social network diversity increased, yet the total number of network members wasn't directly related to the risk of infection. However, compared to those reporting six or more types of social relationships, those reporting just one to three types of social relationships had more than four times the risk of infection. The risk of infection also increased for subjects who exercised two or fewer times per week and those who slept poorly. Subjects with more diverse social connections, greater exercise, and better sleep had greater resistance to the common cold[26].

Reduced stress

Stress predicts mortality. A study in Sweden addressed whether the negative effects of stress could be ameliorated by high levels of social support. Researchers drew a random sample of 752 men who were born in 1933 and living in Gothenburg, Sweden. At baseline, the average age was 50 years. Social support reflected deep emotional relationships and social integration. Seven years post-baseline, 11 percent of the men who self-reported three or more out of ten adverse life events in the year prior to baseline had died compared to 3 percent of the men who reported no adverse life events. Examples of these life events include death of a family member, divorce or separation, and serious financial trouble. However, the relationship between adverse life events and mortality held only for men with low emotional support. Thus, it appears that strong emotional support buffers the adverse effects of stressful life events, especially for men with limited social support[27].

Greater cognitive function in old age

In a unique opportunity for researchers to investigate the risk factors for cognitive impairment in old age, more than 1,100 people from northeastern Illinois agreed to donate their brains to science upon death for the Rush Memory and Aging Project. Prior to death, 89 participants underwent annual clinical evaluations of social networks and cognitive ability. Brains of the deceased were examined for Alzheimer's disease, plus amyloid plaques and tau tangles—both markers of diminished cognitive function. Even at higher levels of brain disease, persons with larger social networks had higher cognitive function. Therefore, social networks may modify the negative effects of brain pathology on cognitive function, consistent with the idea that social networks help individuals create cognitive reserves[28].

Greater likelihood of post-traumatic growth

Post-traumatic growth is defined as "the experience of positive change that occurs as a result of the struggle with highly challenging life crises"[29]. At some point in life, most of us will experience a traumatic event, such as a major accident or illness or loss of a loved one. It turns out that social support and coping strategies can not only help us recover from traumatic events, but also help us grow from the experience. An Italian study followed 41 cancer patients for six months. The study focused on avoidance, coping, and different types of social support: (1) perceived availability of support, (2) actual support received, (3) satisfaction with received support, and (4) competence of the caregiver to address the patient's psychological needs of autonomy, competence, and relatedness. Both the presence of autonomy-supportive caregivers and a problem-focused coping strategy significantly predicted greater post-traumatic growth six months later[30].

A more recent study investigated both general and breast cancer-specific social support and stress as predictors of post-traumatic growth and well-being of breast cancer survivors. The subjects included 173 women (mean age 55) who had recently finished breast cancer treatment. Researchers found that breast cancer-specific social support and breast cancer-specific stress predicted increased levels of post-traumatic growth. Higher levels of general social support and lower levels of general stress both predicted improved well-being. Social support predicted post-traumatic growth and improved well-being in breast cancer survivors[31].

Poor Outcomes Linked to Failing to *Cultivate Social Connections*

People who fail to *Cultivate Social Connections* with family, friends, and their community tend to have shorter lives and experience more physical and mental health problems than people who assiduously *Cultivate Social Connections*. Accumulating evidence points toward perceived social isolation (otherwise known as loneliness) as a major public health threat that predicts increased risks of physical and mental illness and even premature death[32].

Poor Outcomes Linked to Failing to *Cultivate Social Connections*

- Premature death
- Cardiovascular disease
- Dementia
- Longer recover time following surgery
- Poor health
- Faster rate of biological aging
- Greater risk of hospitalization
- Insufficient meaning in life

Premature death

Social isolation is widely believed to be undesirable for most people. Now, a recent study reveals that social isolation is more than simply undesirable—it might shorten life. The English Longitudinal Study of Aging followed 6,500 men and women over age 52 for seven years to evaluate the association of social isolation and loneliness with mortality. Researchers compared the risk of dying during the seven-year follow-up period for persons who displayed the highest and lowest levels of social isolation and loneliness. Social isolation but not loneliness (defined as perceived social isolation) predicted higher risk of premature death for both men and women. The risk of dying for the most socially isolated people, compared to the least socially isolated, ranged from 20-56 percent higher, depending on which confounding factors (such as age, sex, demographic factors) were included in the analyses[33].

Older persons commonly experience loneliness, which can cause distress and impair activities of daily living. While a considerable body of literature exists regarding the effects of social support upon health, fewer studies address the related but distinct topic of loneliness. In one such study, researchers used data from 1,064 participants over age 60 in the Health and Retirement Study. Loneliness was evaluated as feeling left out, feeling isolated, and lacking companionship. Loneliness was associated with the risk of death over the six-year follow-up period. Lonely participants had a 45 percent higher risk of death during follow-up than participants with adequate social support and/or connection. Being lonely predicted significantly increased risks of decline in activities of daily living (59 percent), upper extremities tasks (28 percent), and stair climbing (31 percent). Loneliness might lead to poorer health due to increased inflammation, decreased sleep, and less adherence to medical recommendations[34]. Health outcomes for older people would likely improve with greater social involvement, particularly by developing and maintaining rewarding personal relationships.

Loneliness is a common and serious public health concern, especially for older people. Feelings of distress can arise from discrepancies between one's actual and desired social relationships. Researchers sought to determine if social relationships, health behaviors, and health outcomes affected the link between loneliness and mortality. Research subjects included participants in the National Health and Retirement Study. Subjects who reported feeling lonely in 2002 had a 14 percent higher risk of dying over the next six years than those who reported not feeling lonely. Incorporating social relationships, sleep quality, exercise, and smoking in the statistical model caused the risk to drop by only two percentage points. Thus, loneliness independently predicted a greater risk of premature death. Older adults with the highest levels of loneliness showed a 96 percent higher risk of dying over the six-year follow-up compared to those with the lowest levels of loneliness. Feelings of loneliness appeared to reduce physical and emotional health, thereby leading to a higher risk of dying prematurely. Loneliness may affect our physiology at a basic level. Mechanisms might include increased vascular resistance, increased systolic blood pressure, or reduced immune response[35]. But if we *Cultivate Social Connections*, we may reduce our risk of premature death and increase our *Quality of Lifespan*.

Social isolation—both perceived and actual—predicts an increased risk of premature death and mimics other well-established risk factors for premature mortality. A recent meta-analysis found that social isolation, loneliness, and living alone were associated with a 29, 26, and 32 percent increased risks of mortality, respectively. Moreover, social deficits predicted a higher risk of premature death of subjects younger than age 65[36].

Cardiovascular disease

Stroke is a leading cause of disability and death in the U.S. The lack of perceived neighborhood social cohesion predicts a greater risk of stroke above and beyond traditional risk factors. The eighth wave of the Health and Retirement Study in 2006 addressed several psychological factors for the first time. Participants chose from one of four items that reflected how they perceived social cohesion and social trust in their neighborhoods: (1) I really feel part of this area. (2) Most of the people in this area can be trusted. (3) If you were in trouble, there are lots of people in this area who would help you. (4) Most people in this area are friendly. Of the 6,740 study participants, 265 had a stroke within the four years of follow-up. After controlling for age, gender, chronic illnesses, marital status, education, and total wealth, subjects with a higher perceived social neighborhood cohesion had a 15 percent lower risk of having a stroke[37].

A recent review of articles published between 2002 and 2012 evaluated the relationship between social support, depression, and coronary heart disease. Of the five articles that met the criteria for the review, three found that low social support/being unmarried and depression were independent risk factors for poor cardiac prognosis. Improving the extent and quality of social networks could help cardiac patients, especially those with depression, make healthy choices[38].

Another more recent review and meta-analysis of 23 longitudinal studies in developed countries found that poor social relationships predicted a 29 and 32 percent increase in the incidence of coronary heart disease and stroke, respectively. The increased risks were comparable to those reported in previous research for anxiety and job strain[39]. Social isolation and loneliness may contribute substantially to the disease burden in high-income countries, like the U.S. If we adopt the healthy choice of *Cultivate Social Connections*, we'll likely reduce our risk of being socially isolated or lonely, thereby reducing our risk of cardiovascular disease and stroke.

Dementia

The Kungsholmen Project, a Swedish study, recruited 1,203 non-demented, community-dwelling residents of Stockholm, age 75 or older, with good mental faculties. After three years, researchers found that, compared to married people living with someone, those who were single and lived alone had a 90 percent higher risk of developing dementia. Compared to those with daily to weekly satisfying contacts, those who had no friends or relatives had a 60 percent higher risk of dementia. Compared to people who have daily to weekly satisfying contacts with children, those who have daily to weekly unsatisfying contacts with children showed a 100 percent higher risk of dementia. A composite index of social network showed a graded, increasing risk of dementia as the social network diminished from extensive to moderate to limited to poor. The risk of dementia was 8.26 (!) times higher for people in the "poor" category compared to those in the "extensive" category[40]. Thus, we'll likely reduce our risk of dementia if we *Cultivate Social Connections*.

Epidemiological studies suggest that people with many social contacts, satisfying social relationships, and productive or stimulating cognitive activities have a lower risk of late-life cognitive decline. However, these studies previously suffered from short follow-up periods. To address this defect, researchers in Hawaii used data from 2,513 Japanese American men who participated in the Honolulu Heart Study and the Honolulu-Asia Aging Study; both studies began in 1961. Social engagement was evaluated in 1968 (mid-life) and in 1991 (late-life). Dementia was diagnosed in 1994 and 1997. Compared to men who had high social engagement in both mid- and late life, the risk of dementia for men whose social engagement declined from mid- to late life was 1.87 times higher. Men in the lowest quartile of social engagement in late life had a 2.34 times higher risk of dementia than men in the highest quartile. Low levels of social engagement over the life span or declining levels from mid- to late life may increase our risk of cognitive decline late in life[41].

Longer recovery time following surgery

Six hundred and five mostly male veterans with a mean age of 64 years who were recovering from major thoracic or abdominal operations participated in a randomized controlled trial of massage as a complementary treatment for post-operative pain. The subjects' social networks were assessed by the numbers of friends or relatives each individual had and how frequently the veterans contacted members of their social network. Smaller social network size was associated with a longer hospital stay after surgery. The effect of social networks on surgical outcomes may be mediated by the networks' effect on levels of preoperative pain and anxiety[42].

Poor health

Since parents usually provide meaningful social support for their children, would perceptions of parental caring, and parental loving itself, affect biological and psychological health and illness years later? In the early 1950s, a sample of healthy Harvard undergraduate men who participated in the Harvard Mastery of Stress Study provided ratings of their perceptions of the parental caring they experienced as children. These subjects were followed for 35 years. At midlife, the subjects who suffered from coronary artery disease, hypertension, duodenal ulcer, and alcoholism, among other conditions, gave their parents significantly lower ratings on perceived parental caring items (being loving, just, fair, hardworking, clever, strong) while in college. This effect was independent of the subjects' age, family history of illness, smoking behavior, the death and/or divorce of parents, and marital history of the subjects. Furthermore, 87 percent of subjects who rated both their mother and father as low in parental caring had diagnosed diseases in midlife, whereas only 25 percent of subjects who rated both their mother and father as high in parental caring had diagnosed diseases in midlife. Amazingly, the perception of parental caring on the part of college undergraduates predicted their health 35 years later[43].

Faster rate of biological aging

Loneliness researchers Louise Hawkley and John Cacioppo proposed that loneliness accelerates the rate of age-related declines in physiological regulation and resilience. Several possible pathways include making fewer healthy choices, exposure to stressors, perceived stress, stress response, and the reduced ability to recuperate from stress[44].

Greater risk of hospitalization

The Veterans Aging Cohort Study (VACS) is a longitudinal study of HIV positive and uninfected military veterans at eight VA medical centers nationally. From 2002 to 2008, California researchers followed 1,836 veterans aged 55 and older, with and without HIV, to compare their levels of social isolation and to investigate links with hospital admission and mortality. A Social Isolation Score (SIS) was derived from survey responses about their relationship status, number of friends/family and frequency of visits, involvement in volunteer work, religious activities, self-help groups, or other community activities. The SIS was higher (more isolation) for HIV-positive patients than uninfected patients. The difference increased with age. Social isolation was significantly more prevalent for HIV-positive patients (59 percent) compared to uninfected patients (51 percent). Using pooled data for all patients, social isolation predicted a 25 percent higher risk of hospitalization and a 28 percent higher risk of dying during follow-up of at least two years. The oldest HIV-positive veterans were at especially high risk for hospitalization and death[45].

Another study found that social isolation among older people in Los Angeles predicted a four-fold increase in hospital readmissions over six years. Given the rising proportion of seniors in the U.S. population and the high cost of hospitalizations, group interventions might be a cost-effective way to reduce readmissions and improve people's lives[46].

Insufficient meaning in life

Humans have an innate need for social contact, which provides a route by which we create meaning in our lives. Renowned psychologist Roy Baumeister at Florida State University proposed four criteria for a meaningful life: (1) a sense of purpose, (2) a sense of self-efficacy, (3) the feeling that one's actions have value, and (4) feelings of positive self-worth. Thus, social exclusion should diminish meaning in life. Baumeister and colleagues conducted four experiments with undergraduate students to test whether social exclusion decreased their perceptions of meaning in life[47].

In the first study, students watched a short video featuring an ostensible partner thought to be another undergrad of the same gender (but who was really a researcher). After watching this video, the subjects were told to make their own short video based on the questions that were answered in the previous video. Subjects were randomly assigned to one of three groups that received either (1) rejecting feedback, (2) neutral feedback, or (3) accepting feedback from their ostensible partner.

Study two was similar conceptually, but used the interactive, ball-throwing computer game Cyberball. During the game, subjects thought they were playing with three other persons, but in reality were playing against the computer. Subjects were randomly assigned to one of three groups: (1) ostracism, (2) control, and (3) high inclusion. The subjects in the high-inclusion group controlled the ball the most, while those in the ostracism group controlled the ball the least. At the beginning of each study, students filled out questionnaires that measured meaningfulness and meaninglessness. For studies one and two, researchers found that subjects in the rejection and ostracism groups reported lower meaningfulness and higher meaninglessness, respectively.

In the third study, undergrads filled out questionnaires that measured meaningfulness, social exclusion, depression, happiness, optimism, and mood. The presence of greater meaning in a student's life predicted significantly lower loneliness and depression, and significantly predicted greater happiness, optimism, and mood. Of these, loneliness most strongly predicted less meaning in life.

In study four, undergrads filled out questionnaires that measured meaningfulness, social exclusion, plus Baumeister's four aspects of meaning (purpose, self-efficacy, value, and self-worth). As expected, all four aspects of meaning affected the relationship between meaningfulness and social exclusion.

Taken together, the four studies suggest that rejection and loneliness are associated with low meaning in life. Social exclusion diminishes the four aspects that define meaning in life[48]. These studies illustrate benefits of making the healthy choice *Cultivate Social Connections* a key aspect of everyday life.

Practical Ways to *Cultivate Social Connections*

- **Volunteer for a community organization.** It should be easy to find an organization that you would like to support with your time and energy. Volunteering will help you cultivate social connections and build community. Your town may have a register of local organizations that need volunteer help. Examples abound. Consider trading an hour a week of web surfing or TV viewing for an hour of volunteering every week. You'd get the benefits of less sitting, moving around more, and cultivating social connections.

- **Share your sorrows with other people.** Large surveys of corporate employees and college students show that the more friends we have, the healthier you are. The benefit is due, almost entirely, to the degree to which we talk to our friends about the traumatic events in your life. If you have had a major upheaval in your life and have supportive friends, talk about it. Simply having friends is not enough[49].

- **Learn to be fully present with others.** Matt Tenney's book *Mindfulness Edge* offers useful suggestions to improve mindfulness in your daily life. Several of Tenney's suggestions can also help you cultivate social support. A bedrock purpose of mindfulness is to serve others. One key aspect of serving is to be fully present in all encounters with other people. Being fully present increases your empathy with others. Being present helps you meet everyone with an attitude of agape love (reflecting a sense of benevolent goodwill). People want to be seen and heard. Being present shows other people that you care about them, increasing the likelihood that they will care about you[50]. Being mindful helps you *Cultivate Social Connections.*

- **Improve your listening skills.** Listening is critical for forming and maintaining strong, healthy social relationships. Careful listening acknowledges the value of another and allows people to feel that they are being heard. Everyone has a fundamental need for expression and recognition. Listening well requires you to let go of what's on your mind long enough to hear the other person's concerns. Unfortunately, you may often fail to resist the impulse to provide advice or argue, rather than simply hearing what the other person has to say. In his eminently readable book *The Lost Art of Listening,* psychologist Michael Nichols provides a compelling account of the importance of listening and how you can develop better listener skills[51]. I recommend it highly.

Three Key Points

1. *Cultivating Social Connections* may be the single most important thing you can do to create lifelong vibrant health and emotional well-being.

2. Social connections help create meaning in your life and help prevent feelings of isolation and loneliness.

3. The social support that you give to others probably provides greater health benefits for you than the support you receive from others.

Chapter 5

Defuse Chronic Stress

*The greatest weapon against stress is our ability
to choose one thought over another.*
—William James

We've all heard a lot about stress, mainly about how bad it is. But what is stress, anyway? Psychologists often define stress as having three characteristics: (1) a measurable arousal response, (2) something perceived as negative, and (3) the subject perceiving a lack of control over the stressor[1]. According to this definition, a particular event—such as being asked to give a public speech—may or may not be a stressor. Some people do not perceive giving a speech in a negative light or feel a lack of control when speaking publicly. It's important to remember this definition when reading accounts of the impacts of "stressful" situations. By this definition, some "stress" may not be bad.

Two Kinds of Stress

There are generally two kinds of stress: acute and chronic. Acute stress, also known as the "fight-or-flight response," evolved as a survival mechanism. It operates over a short period of time. Acute stress triggers a surge of hormones to help us either deal with the perceived threat or flee to safety. Examples of acute stressors include having a job interview, narrowly avoiding a car accident, or encountering a barking dog while jogging. Chronic stress, like an ongoing worry or hassle, occurs more frequently. For example, a high-pressure job, a divorce, or commuting to work in heavy traffic twice a day can be highly stressful. Chronic stressors stimulate the prolonged production of stress hormones, including cortisol. Over time, these hormones induce a cascade of damaging effects on our body, the cost of which is referred to as "allostatic load." The combination of chronic stress, a sedentary lifestyle, and eating poor-quality food can lead to increased secretions of additional hormones that, along with insulin, promote the deposition of body fat, the formation of arterial plaques, the alteration of brain function, and impaired immunity. If we learn to *Defuse Chronic Stress,* we can greatly improve our physical and psychological health[2].

Allostatic load refers to the cumulative physiological damage that results from allostatic (stability-seeking) responses of the body to chronic stressors.

Dozens of peer-reviewed publications during the last century show that the "relaxation response" and other mind-body practices effectively treat a variety of stress-related conditions. These include chronic insomnia, diabetes, arthritis, recovery from surgery, infertility, premenstrual syndrome, menopausal hot flashes, and nausea from chemotherapy. In fact, mind-body practices (such as meditation, mindfulness, tai chi, yoga, and guided imagery) have been found to be equally if not more effective in treating chronic insomnia than medications. Mind-body interventions have the important added benefit of improving our sense of self-control and self-confidence, which can help us incorporate healthy behaviors into our daily life. Such interventions dampen the sympathetic nervous system, which triggers the fight-or-flight response (characterized by rapid heartbeat and breathing, among other physical changes). Interventions may activate the parasympathetic nervous system, which acts like a brake to help our body calm down[3].

Chronic stress is linked to major chronic diseases including clinical depression, cardiovascular disease, HIV/AIDS, and cancer. In medical literature, chronic stress is frequently associated with upper respiratory infections, asthma, herpes infections, autoimmune disorders, and wound healing. The consistency of the research strongly supports a causal link between psychological stress and disease[4].

Chronic stress early in life, especially for children in low-socio-economic circumstances and in harsh family environments, may compromise key biological systems in ways that reduce their resiliency. Research reveals that low-socioeconomic circumstances in harsh family environments predict increased elevated C-reactive protein (a marker of inflammation) levels and increased blood pressure in adulthood[5].

Benefits Linked to *Defuse Chronic Stress*

We can't avoid stress entirely; it's a normal part of daily life. Sometimes it's even useful. It can help us be more productive and even temporarily boost memory. But chronic stress can wreak havoc on our bodies. However, if we learn to *Defuse Chronic Stress*, we can expect important benefits for our health and well-being, as listed below.

Benefits Linked to *Defuse Chronic Stress*	Improved *Quality of Lifespan* Greater longevity Improved self-control Improved overall health Reduced risk of cancer Greater longevity following cancer diagnosis Better performance in school

Improved *Quality of Lifespan*

Mindfulness-based stress reduction (MBSR) is an effective educational approach that uses mindfulness meditation, yoga, and body awareness to teach people with one or more medical conditions how to take better care of themselves and live healthier, more adaptive lives. But is MSBR beneficial for people who people who don't exhibit a clinical condition? Researchers recently reviewed 29 studies that included 2,688 evidently healthy adults. These studies used MBSR as an intervention to investigate the effects of stress on anxiety and other psychological states. MBSR had large, positive effects on stress generally; moderate effects on anxiety, depression, distress, and quality of life; and small effects on burnout. Together, changes in mindfulness and measures of compassion correlated with changes in the clinical measures of stress immediately post-treatment and at follow-up. The researchers concluded that MBSR is, in fact, "moderately effective in reducing stress, depression, anxiety and distress, and in improving the quality of life of healthy individuals[6]".

Greater longevity

It's widely understood that prolonged psychological stress contributes to high blood pressure and heart disease. Stress reduction through Transcendental Meditation (TM), a simple technique practiced twice a day for 20 minutes, has been shown to reduce blood pressure in persons with clinical conditions, such as hypertension. Researchers used data from two randomized controlled trials with 202 hypertensive subjects (mean age 72 years at baseline); the average follow-up time was nearly 8 years. The trials compared the effects of TM with other stress-reduction techniques. Subjects in the combined TM groups had a statistically significant 23 percent lower risk of mortality over the follow-up period compared to combined subjects in the mindfulness training, mental relaxation, and usual care groups. Similarly, subjects in the TM groups had a statistically significant 30 percent lower risk of cardiovascular mortality. Interestingly, the subjects in the two TM trials were quite different: white and primarily female living in homes for the elderly in the Boston area in one, and community-dwelling African American men and women in Oakland, California, in the other. The large difference between the groups of subjects suggests that the results of the analysis may apply to other populations of older, hypertensive people as well[7].

Improved self-control

People who believe they have control over their lives tend to make more healthful choices than people who don't. It's the belief rather than the actual fact of control that matters. A sense of control helps us respond deliberately rather than instinctively to stressful situations. For example, a sense of control helps our brain inhibit the reward-seeking behavior that comes instinctively from reacting to hunger. When we're hungry but also feel in control of our life, we are more able to resist the need for immediate hunger relief at a fast food outlet, thus making a decision that's more aligned with our long-term goals. If we're driving, we might continue home and eat a handful of almonds instead of inhaling a 1,460-calorie burger at a fast-food joint[8].

How often and how strongly do we experience desires, and to what extent do our desires conflict with our goals? To investigate desires and our attempts to control them, researchers conducted a large study based on integrating desire strength, conflict, resistance (self-control), and behavior enactment. More than 200 adults wore beepers for a week and furnished 7,827 reports of desire episodes. Results suggested that desires were frequent, variable in intensity, and largely unproblematic. Urges that *did* conflict with the subjects' goals tended to elicit resistance, with uneven success. Desire strength, conflict, resistance, and self-regulatory success were influenced by personality variables, as well as by situational and interpersonal factors. These include alcohol use, the mere presence of others, and the presence of others who already enacted the desire in question. Whereas personality variables had a stronger impact on dimensions of desire (desire strength and conflict) that emerged early, situational factors (resistance and behavior enactment) showed more influence on dimensions of desire later[9]. The practical message of this study: Avoid situations that are likely to create a stress response. For example, don't shop at the grocery store when you're tired and hungry.

Improved overall health

Until recently, most researchers thought that most chronic conditions began in adulthood. Thus, health authorities largely directed preventive measures toward adults. Accumulating evidence now reveals that at least some chronic conditions begin in childhood. Compared to children raised in nurturing families and who experience minimal youthful chronic stress, children

Mind-Body Interventions Reduce Medical Costs

Health care expenditures for stress-related disorders rank the third highest in the U.S. behind heart disease and cancer. Researchers in Boston wanted to know whether mind-body interventions could impact the demand for and costs of medical services. The researchers used data from the Benson-Henry Institute to answer this question. Subjects included those who sought care at the Institute from January 12, 2006, through July 1, 2014, and who underwent the Relaxation Response Resiliency Program (3RP) during the study period. The 3RP program included relaxation-response-eliciting meditation and mindfulness exercises, social support, cognitive skills training, and positive psychology. (This program incorporated four of the healthy lifestyle choices– *Cultivate Social Connections, Defuse Chronic Stress, Keep Learning, Develop a Positive Mental Attitude*–this book promotes.) The overall outcome for health-resource utilization was billable encounters and their associated services. The period for the study started one year prior to the intervention and ran until the intervention ended. For the control group, which contained individuals raised in dysfunctional families and who experience chronic stress during childhood have a higher risk of illness and premature death. Two mechanisms might account for these findings. First, chronic stress in childhood may disrupt physiological processes, leading to damage that accumulates over time, thereby increasing allostatic load. Second, stress may cause adverse physiological and physical changes, especially in the brain, that persist but do not manifest until adulthood. Adverse effects of chronic stress in childhood probably account for some of the underperformance of disadvantaged children in school and their difficulty adapting resourcefully to life as adults. If future research confirms the present findings, the implications for public health policy could be enormous. Early childhood programs such as Head Start could be reconfigured to help reduce chronic stress that disadvantaged kids experience. Reducing chronic stress might improve academic performance and lead to better health both during childhood and adulthood[10].

matched to the intervention group in terms of age, gender, and ethnicity, the study period ran backward for one year ("pre" intervention) and forward one year ("post" intervention) from the midpoint of their time in the health care system.

For patients in the 3RP intervention group and for patients that highly utilized health care, total resources (clinical, imaging, laboratory, and procedures) declined significantly from before to after participation in the 3RP intervention. For the control group, none of the comparable resource utilizations declined significantly. Rough estimates indicated that the 3RP would pay for itself in four to six months by avoiding emergency room costs alone, not to mention other treatment costs[11].

The benefits of 3RP and other mindfulness programs align with the nascent shift in medical care from high use of specialized care for late-term disease to patient-centered approaches that promote wellness, support self-care, provide preventive care, and manage diseases.

Reduced risk of cancer

In chapter 1, we looked at how *shinrin-yoku*, or forest bathing, helps reduce stress. Shinrin-yoku might also improve our immune system by increasing the activity of both natural killer cells (which induce tumor cell death) and proportions of natural killer, T cells, and proteins (which have anti-cancer activity). In one study, 12 apparently healthy men (mean age 43 years) spent three nights and two days in two forests. A variety of samples and measurements were taken from the subjects (including blood samples, a mood states questionnaire, activity using a pedometer, and sleep) during a typical day at work before the forest visit, during the visit, and immediately afterwards. Eleven of the 12 subjects showed higher natural killer cell activity after the forest visit compared to before the forest visit. Forest bathing itself also increased the number of natural killer cells and other anti-cancer cells and proteins[12]. Frequent visits to a forest might reduce our risk of cancer by helping us *Defuse Chronic Stress*.

Greater longevity following cancer diagnosis

Cancer exacts an enormous psychological and physical toll globally. Psychological interventions can improve cancer patients' mental outlook. Some evidence suggests that interventions can also extend survival after diagnosis and surgery for patients with early stage malignant melanoma. One intervention included structured group meetings in which 68 malignant melanoma patients met weekly for 1.5 hours for six weeks. The content of the meetings included health education, stress management, enhancement of coping skills, and psychological support from other patients and program staff. An analysis at 10 years post-intervention showed that patients in the intervention group had a statistically greater likelihood of survival and a longer recurrence-free period from cancer than those in the typical care group, regardless of patients' age, gender, and tumor thickness and location[13]. If we learn to *Defuse Chronic Stress*, we may live longer, even with a cancer diagnosis.

Better performance in school

The feeling of being an outsider can create chronic stress that leads to reduced performance and poorer health. A recent study investigated a psychological intervention designed to help African-American college freshman undergraduates reframe their stressful thoughts about adversity arising from feeling that they didn't belong at a specific college. Forty-nine African-American and 43 Euro-American students were randomly assigned to either the intervention or a control condition. The intervention lasted for one hour at the beginning of the fall term and encouraged the students to think of adversity as a part of the college adjustment process rather than a fixed deficit unique to them or their ethnic group. Over the course of three years, students who received the intervention increased their perceived sense of belonging, compared to African-American students who didn't receive it or Euro-American students who received the intervention or not. In addition, the African-American students increased their academic performance relative to the Euro-American students; experienced fewer negative racial stereotypes, less self-doubt, and better health; and reported fewer doctor visits in the final month of college, along with greater subjective happiness than the other students[14]. Who would have guessed that the positive effects of a single, one-hour intervention would persist for three years?!

Poor Outcomes Linked to Failing to *Defuse Chronic Stress*

While short-term stress is typically manageable and not likely to cause serious health problems, stress that persists can harm our physical health and emotional well-being. This section discusses problems that can arise from failing to *Defuse Chronic Stress*.

Bad Outcomes Linked to Failing to *Defuse Chronic Stress*
- Premature death
- Cardiovascular disease
- Hypertension
- Dementia and cognitive decline
- Mitochondrial dysfunction
- Shortened telomeres
- Body distress syndrome
- Overeating
- Metabolic syndrome
- Higher work-related costs

Premature death

Because stress can appear in different guises, researchers have devised different ways to measure stress. One area of research focuses on stressful life events (SLE), which include adverse effects for individuals and their loved ones. Examples of SLE include death of a spouse, divorce, and termination at work. Hassles comprise another type of stress, including daily, relatively minor problems that often arise from social relationships, the built environment, and technology. In the following study, chronic stress refers to ongoing problems often linked to social roles, such as troubled marriages and conflicts at work.

Psychologist Carolyn Aldwin and her colleagues wanted to know if hassles changed the effects of stressful life events on the risk of dying prematurely. Study subjects included 1,293 men who enrolled in the Veteran's Administration Normative Aging Study. Between 1961 and 1970, men in the Boston area were screened for good health (lack of chronic diseases or physical disability). The follow-up period ended in 2010, by which time 553 of the 1,293 men had died. Higher mortality was significantly associated with categories of higher stress related to SLE and with a higher intensity of hassles. Additional analysis showed that stressful life events and intense hassles independently predicted a higher risk of dying prematurely[15].

Researchers identified 10 physiological components of allostatic load. These components include systolic and diastolic blood pressure, total cholesterol, and abdominal obesity, among others. The researchers obtained data from 1,189 participants aged 70–79 in the Established Populations for Epidemiological Studies of the Elderly to see if allostatic load (scored from 0 to 10) predicted risk of mortality, cardiovascular disease, physical function, and cognitive function over an 8-year follow-up period. Mortality risk increased significantly as allostatic load increased. Participants with scores of seven or greater had a 542 percent higher risk of death compared to participants who had scores of zero—that's a huge difference! Physical function and cognitive function both declined significantly as allostatic load increased. This finding was even

Our Perception of Stress Affects Mortality Risk

Researchers at the University of Wisconsin used data from the 1998 National Health Interview Survey to investigate the relationship between the amount of stress that people experience, their perception of that stress, and how those factors affect the risk of dying prematurely. The survey collected information from 28,753 people who formed a representative cross-section of Americans. At the beginning of the study, people who reported that stress affected their health to some degree or a lot had an 80 and 326 percent higher risk of self-reporting poor health, respectively, compared to those who reported that stress had hardly any or no effect on their health. But here's the kicker: While neither the amount of stress nor the perception of stress independently predicted mortality after eight years of follow-up, the presence of lots of stress and the perception of the stress as bad increased the risk of mortality by 43 percent.

This important study shows us that it isn't stress as such but our perception of stress that predicts our risk of dying. Our mindset or attitude toward the stressful events in our life can matter more than the events themselves[17].

more impressive given that the study group included only participants in the top one-third of physical and cognitive abilities[16].

Cardiovascular disease

Adverse metabolic changes caused by persistent stress might cause cardiovascular disease. Inflammation of arterial walls and subsequent deposition of LDL-cholesterol particles that form plaque in the artery walls can cause cardiovascular disease. Plaque causes artery walls to narrow, thereby reducing blood flow. Additionally, the stress hormone cortisol is associated with the buildup of calcium in the arteries, which is unhealthy.

A recent literature review showed that chronic stress, both early in life and during adulthood, predicted a 40 and 60 percent increase, respectively, in the risk of cardiovascular disease. Social isolation and loneliness are sources of chronic stress. A meta-analysis of published studies showed that these factors predicted a 50 percent increase in the risk of coronary heart disease. Yet another meta-analysis found that job strain was associated with a 34 percent increase in the risk of coronary heart disease, after adjusting for age and sex. Taken together, these and other studies support the idea that chronic stress is a causal factor in cardiovascular disease[18].

Hypertension

The prevalence of hypertension (high blood pressure) in Americans aged 65 and over jumped from 44 percent in 1993–1995 to 55 percent in 2001–2003. The estimated annual medical costs topped $100 billion. For elderly persons, systolic hypertension is a more important risk factor for cardiovascular disease than either diastolic blood pressure or excessive blood lipids (such as cholesterol and triglycerides).

Drug therapies for systolic hypertension often have side effects. Thus, safe and effective non-drug therapies are important. Stress-management techniques that elicit the relaxation response reduce the risk of hypertension. But do they work for elderly persons with systolic hypertension? Researchers studied 122 patients over age 55 with systolic hypertension who were also receiving drug therapy. The patients were randomly assigned to one of two groups: a treatment group that received eight weeks of training in the relaxation response, and a control group that received eight weeks of lifestyle modification. After eight weeks, systolic blood pressure declined by 9.4 and 8.8 mm Hg in the relaxation and lifestyle groups, respectively—with no significance difference between them. However, when 44 of the relaxation-response participants and 36 of the lifestyle-modification participants became eligible for supervised hypertensive drug elimination, patients in the relaxation-response group were 3.3 times more likely to successfully eliminate their medication than patients in the lifestyle group. Thus, failing to *Defuse Chronic Stress* can lead to higher blood pressure, while missing a golden opportunity to reduce blood pressure into a safe range and potentially eliminate the need for drug therapy[19].

In a large review of stress-reduction and high blood pressure studies involving 960 participants and 23 treatment comparisons, Transcendental Meditation showed large and statistically significant declines in systolic/diastolic blood pressure (−5.0/−2.8 mm Hg), while biofeedback (−0.8/−2.0 mm Hg); relaxation-assisted progressive muscle relaxation (-1.9/−1.4 mm Hg); and stress management training (−2.3/−1.3 mm Hg) did not[20].

Dementia and cognitive decline

The World Health Organization[21] estimated that the number of patients with dementia will triple worldwide from 2010 to 2050. Because chronic distress is potentially modifiable, researchers seek to understand the mechanism(s) by which chronic distress might affect cognition later in life. One possible mechanism is chronic stress that leads to brain pathology, which then leads to cognitive problems. Researchers used data from the Religious Orders Study over a 10-year period to investigate this idea. Two hundred nineteen participants were older Catholic nuns, priests, and brothers who agreed to annual clinical evaluations (including neurological examination and cognitive testing) and whose brains were autopsied upon death. Researchers found that the risk of dementia near the time of death increased by 53 percent for each one-point increase (on a scale from 0-20) in a composite measure of chronic distress. A person in the highest 10 percent of distress had twice the risk of dementia compared to a person in the lowest 10 percent of distress. Chronic distress was associated with an increased risk of dementia and reduced cognition—but curiously not to the leading causes of neuropathology—such as neurofibrillary tangles, cerebral infarctions, and the beta-amyloid peptide. This unexpected result suggests the presence of a novel mechanism that regulates stress-related behavior and memory[22].

Other evidence suggests that cognitive training and lifestyle choices might forestall or even reverse dementia. Meditation could be regarded as one form of cognitive training. Recent research suggests that meditation is associated with a reduced rate of cognitive decline with age. Longitudinal studies have found beneficial effects of meditation on age-related cognitive performance, cognitive flexibility, task switching, memory verbal fluency, and attention. A large body of evidence suggests that meditation helps *Defuse Chronic Stress*.

Meditation appears to be worthwhile for this purpose alone. Yet no consensus exists with respect to which meditation approach might provide the greatest stream of cognitive benefits[23].

Mitochondrial dysfunction

Mitochondria are structures in cells that break down carbohydrates and fatty acids to liberate energy. A recent review sheds light on how chronic stress may promote mitochondrial dysfunction. Chronically elevated levels of blood glucose damage both mitochondria and mitochondrial DNA. Damage can include toxic products that promote inflammation, change gene expression, and promote cell aging. The cumulative damage to mitochondria is thought to occur through this sequence of events[24].

1. Chronic stress, inactivity, and overeating elevate both stress hormones and blood glucose, and collectively promote insulin resistance.

2. Insulin resistance leads to mitochondrial damage, causing fragmentation, degraded mitochondrial quality, and increased levels of harmful free radicals.

3. Mitochondrial damage in turn leads to cellular dysfunction and mitochondrial aging.

4. Organ and systems failure ensue, which manifest as high blood pressure, cardiovascular disease, type 2 diabetes, neurodegeneration, plus physical and cognitive decline.

On the bright side, healthy lifestyle choices, especially *Keep Moving, Eat Better,* and *Defuse Chronic Stress,* may help protect us from this highly undesirable chain of events.

Shortened telomeres

Psychological stress leads to shorter telomeres (the protective caps on the ends of chromosomes) and less telomerase (an enzyme that lengthens telomeres). Over time, as cells divide, telomeres become shorter and shorter until they are so short that cell division stops. Shorter telomeres are associated with cellular aging.

Women with chronically ill children would presumably experience more chronic stress than women with healthy children. Would women with chronically ill kids have shorter telomeres? To test this idea, researchers enrolled 58 healthy, premenopausal women in a study. Nineteen of the mothers had healthy children, while 39 had a chronically ill child. The researchers found that both perceived stress and longer stress duration were associated with shorter telomere length, lower telomerase activity, and higher oxidative stress. In this study, the highest-stressed women had shorter telomeres corresponding to 9–17 years of increased biological age compared to the lowest-stressed women. (A previous study showed that shorter telomere length is associated with higher mortality rates in older people.) Therefore, learning to *Defuse Chronic Stress* may have a major positive impact on our long-term health and well-being[25].

Body distress syndrome

Bodily distress syndrome (BDS) is an umbrella diagnosis for conditions with bothersome, unexplained physical symptoms, including fibromyalgia, irritable bowel syndrome, and chronic fatigue syndrome. BDS accounts for 20–35 percent of medical care consultations in the Netherlands. Effective treatment is difficult to achieve. To learn whether mindfulness therapy would be superior to enhanced standard treatment of BDS, Danish researchers randomized 119 patients to either 1) mindfulness-based stress reduction with some cognitive behavioral therapy elements, or 2) enhanced standard treatment that included two-hour specialist medical care and brief cognitive behavioral therapy. The study showed that both approaches improved physical health from baseline to follow-up 15 months later. Nevertheless, the mindfulness therapy group improved earlier in the 15-month treatment period, while the enhanced usual treatment group improved later[26].

The Danish researchers also estimated the economic consequences of the mindfulness and enhanced usual treatment interventions. After 15 months, 25 percent of the mindfulness group received a disability pension compared to 44 percent of the enhanced usual treatment group. Total health care costs, including the costs of both interventions, declined for both groups combined, from a median of $2,971 pre-treatment to $1,593 post-treatment (expressed in 2007 U.S. dollars). Thus, mindfulness intervention reduced both the rate of BDS patients receiving a disability pension and overall medical care costs[27].

Overeating

Chronic psychological stress may contribute to abdominal fat from external-based and emotional eating. Abdominal fat produces inflammation, which in turn promotes insulin resistance and metabolic syndrome. Researchers in California tested whether mindfulness training would reduce psychological stress, leading to reduced emotional eating and less abdominal fat. Forty-seven overweight or obese women participated in the study. Those in the treatment group received nine, 2.5-hour mindfulness training sessions over four months and one seven-hour guided meditation. The control group consisted of wait-listed participants. The researchers found that those in the treatment group reported significantly greater increases on three of the four mindfulness scales than those in the control group. Those in the treatment group also reported significantly lower anxiety. Both groups reported lower levels of external-based and emotional eating, but the treatment group showed significantly greater improvement. The two groups did not differ greatly over four months in terms of body weight or abdominal fat. Increases in responsiveness to bodily sensations and decreases in chronic stress were significantly related to greater declines in abdominal fat but only for the treatment group. Cortisol response was significantly lower for obese participants in the treatment group, but not in the control group. While the mindfulness training group members overall did not reduce caloric intake, those in the mindfulness group who increased mindfulness, decreased chronic stress, and decreased emotional eating did reduce their abdominal fat[28].

Metabolic syndrome

Stress at work may increase the risk of cardiovascular disease by promoting metabolic syndrome—a group of conditions that includes high abdominal obesity, high blood triglycerides, high blood pressure, and high fasting glucose. One British study tested 10,308 civil service employees in London to see whether work stress was associated with the presence of metabolic syndrome. Chronic work stress was defined as employees reporting high job demands and low job control on three of four questionnaires administered during 14 years of follow-up. Compared to employees without chronic work stress, employees with chronic work stress had a 139 percent higher risk of having metabolic syndrome at the end of follow-up. The risk increased in a dose-response manner as the number of times employees reported high job demand and low job control increased from zero to four[29].

Higher work-related costs

The American Institute of Stress reported that roughly 60 percent of doctor visits stem from stress-related complaints and illnesses. Chronic stress as it affects workplace health and well-being is no minor matter. In total, American businesses lose $300 billion annually to lowered productivity, absenteeism, and health care costs stemming from stress[30].

Practical Ways to *Defuse Chronic Stress*

The consequences of chronic stress can be serious, affecting both our psychological and physical well-being. Fortunately, you can try several ways to help manage stress more effectively. According to the American Psychological Association, the best stress-relieving activities include spending time in nature, physical exercise, sports, praying, attending a religious service, reading, listening to music, spending time with friends and family, getting a massage, and meditating[31]. Let's look more closely at a few ways to *Defuse Chronic Stress.*

- **Spend time outdoors.** Exposure to nature is associated with many health benefits: reduced stress, reduced blood pressure, lower mortality from cardiovascular disease, better mood, and greater social well-being, among others[32]. Take a walk, eat your lunch on a park bench, head for the hills, ride a bike, look out your window at the greenery, sit by a body of water. Simply get more nature into your life.

- **Develop a stress-enhancing mindset**. In her book *Mindset*, psychologist Carol Dweck explored how our mindset affects our views of and experiences in the world[33]. More recently, Alia Crum and her colleagues extended the concept of mindset as a distinct and meaningful variable that influences stress response. They proposed the idea of a stress mindset as the extent to which a person believes that stress can enhance (the stress-enhancing mindset) or diminish (the stress-debilitating mindset) positive stress-related outcomes such as performance and productivity. Previous work suggested that reframing stress in a positive light is possible and can lead to positive outcomes, at least in certain circumstances. With enhanced awareness, we can be primed to adopt a stress-enhancing mindset that may lead to positive health and better performance outcomes[34].

- **Reappraise stress as excitement.** We often feel anxious when anticipating stressful events such as an annual performance review, public speaking, or taking a test. However, evidence shows that when people are instructed to reframe their anxiety as excitement—in karaoke singing, or public speaking, or solving difficult math problems—they report feeling more excited and perform better than those who are instructed to be calm. The way we talk to ourselves (self-talk) about our feelings influences whether we feel anxious or excited. Anxiety need not be avoided or suppressed (which might not be effective) but can be reappraised as something useful. We can successfully reappraise stress with minimal time and effort, at least in some situations[35].

- **Minimize negative self-talk.** Consider a situation in which an external stressor interferes with life. A "favorite" for me is computer-related problems. Imagine that I'm working on a report that's due tomorrow. I'm pleased that I finished the report a day early. As I start to print the document, my printer suddenly stops working, but I can't figure out what's causing the problem. I feel tension building in my shoulders. At this point, I often descend into a litany of negative self-talk: "What did I do to deserve this? Why does this always happen to me? Why doesn't this printer have a detailed instruction manual? Arrgh!" My negative self-talk magnifies the stress created by the printer malfunction, leading to further negative emotions, which lead to negative behaviors and poor outcomes. Recently, I've become more aware that my negative self-talk makes matters worse. On my better days, I now respond to technological problems with thoughts such as, "Maybe I could copy the file to a thumb drive and take it to an office supply store to be printed. Maybe if I turn off my computer and printer then restart them that will fix things." I realize now that my response to the stressor can either increase or decrease my stress level. Being mindful in the moment, acknowledging the situation, and remembering the ill effects of negative thoughts and self-talk helps me remain calm(er) and respond resourcefully. Positive thoughts can lead to positive emotions, which can lead to positive behaviors and better outcomes.

- **Learn to relax.** Numerous techniques, including guided imagery, breath focus, and the relaxation response are available. Herbert Benson, a pioneer in mind-body medicine, established in the 1970s that our mental state can alter our body's physiological functioning. He coined the term "relaxation response," which refers to our ability to encourage positive changes in our body that make our muscles and organs slow down and enhance blood flow to the brain. The relaxation response is opposite to the stress response. We can facilitate natural recovery from illness by the state of our mind. The relaxation response can be elicited through several meditative and prayer-based techniques[36]. Follow these steps:

The Relaxation Response

1. Find a quiet place and sit in a comfortable position.
2. Focus on a word, phrase, image, or short prayer.
3. Close your eyes.
4. Progressively relax all your muscles for 1–2 minutes.
5. Breathe slowly and naturally; repeat the word or phrase on the exhale.
6. Assume a passive attitude; if thoughts arise, simply let them pass by.
7. Continue the exercise for 12–15 minutes.
8. Practice the technique at least once daily, preferably first thing in the morning or late afternoon.

- **Connect with others.** Helping other people benefits not only the recipients, it benefits us. The Changing Lives of Older Couples study revealed that among older people who provided help to others during the previous year, stress was not associated with an increased risk of dying[37]. While many of us may think that the benefits of helping others apply only to those being helped, this study indicates that the benefits can apply to the persons doing the helping. The healthy choice of *Cultivate Social Connections* may lead us to help others (such as shoveling snow from an elderly neighbor's sidewalk) and, thereby, *Defuse Chronic Stress*.

- **Practice meditation.** Meditation can decrease stress, anxiety, depression, and pain[38]. We can choose from many types of meditation.

- **Practice mindfulness.** People with high levels of mindfulness are more likely to regulate their emotions and more rapidly recover from distress. Similarly, people with high levels of mindfulness are more likely to use their emotions to enhance performance to reduce perceived stress[39]. One simple way to cultivate mindfulness is focus on each moment in our daily life. This approach will help you notice when you're stressed. Then you can take appropriate action.

- **Practice empathic listening.** Clinical psychologist Arthur P. Ciaramicoli presents a compelling case in his book *The Stress Solution: Using Empathy and Cognitive Behavioral Therapy* to reduce anxiety and develop resilience. Dr. Ciaramicoli maintains that poor relationships with others, and the accompanying chronic stress arise from poor communication skills. The key to being a better communicator is learning how to listen to other people while being truly present and non-judgmental. In addition, we must learn to avoid cognitive distortion, such as blaming, mind reading, and projection. I highly recommend buying this book and doing the exercises to reduce your level of chronic stress and bring greater peace to your life.

Three Key Points

1. Chronic psychological stress predicts serious physiological and psychological effects leading to a diminished *Quality of Lifespan* and other ills.

2. Happily, a variety of simple techniques can help *Defuse Chronic Stress*.

3. The positive effects of *Defuse Chronic Stress* can ripple throughout life.

Chapter 6

Keep Learning

In the last two decades, something remarkable has occurred
in relation to lifelong learning; as a concept, it has been
almost universally embraced.[1]
—Stephen Roche

A stimulated, challenged brain not only leads to an enriched life,
and also help stave off physical ailments and diseases as we age.
Our brain is much like our skeletal muscles. We have to work our
muscles to keep them functioning properly. Similarly, we have to keep
using our brain in creative ways to keep it functioning properly. The
saying, "use 'em or lose 'em," applies to the brain's neural connections.
Using our brain through continued learning will help establish and
maintain neural connections that support lifelong vibrant health and
emotional well-being.

Benefits Linked to *Keep Learning*

If we *Keep Learning*, we'll be more likely to maintain sharp mental
faculties for the rest of our lives. The following list captures some of
the benefits we can expect to enjoy if we *Keep Learning*.

	Increased longevity
	Increased health literacy
	Increased cognitive reserve
Benefits Linked to	Reduced risk of dementia and cognitive decline
Keep Learning	Increased goal-directed activity
	Development of new life skills
	Improved balance
	Improved growth mindset

Increased longevity

Reading this book might help you live longer! Researchers at Yale University used book and periodical reading data from 3,645 individuals in the Health and Retirement Study. Participants, who were followed for an average of nine years, were grouped into three categories according to how many hours per week they reported reading books (0, 0.01–3.49, or more than 3.49) or periodicals (0–2, 2.01–6.99, or more than 6.99). Compared to those in the lowest one-third of book reading hours, participants in the highest one-third of book reading had a 23 percent lower risk of dying during the study, after adjusting for confounding factors such as age and education. The survival advantage for periodical readers was lower than for book readers. When book reading was collapsed into two groups—zero vs. some reading—book readers enjoyed a 23-month survival advantage[2].

Book reading is one of the most accessible and potentially valuable ways to *Keep Learning*. Given that Americans over age 65 spend an average of 4.4 hours a day watching TV, switching one of those hours to reading a book might increase longevity and *Quality of Lifespan*.

Increased health literacy

The healthy lifestyle choice *Keep Learning*, based on the premise of "use it or lose it," aims to keep our brain active. However, another important benefit of lifelong learning is acquiring important, health-related information. Learning includes reading and correctly interpreting medication labels. Researchers have long known that a person's educational level is highly correlated with longevity. Reading fluency may partially account for this association. People who are good readers are more likely than poor readers to be aware of appropriate self-care strategies and can better understand written instructions from health care providers.

Researchers recruited 3,260 new Medicare recipients to determine if those with low health literacy died earlier than those with high health literacy. At the end of the study's six-year follow-up, participants with inadequate health literacy had a 52 percent higher risk of mortality than those with adequate health literacy. Most of the excess mortality arose from cardiovascular deaths. Thus, improved health literacy might help us live longer and better[3].

Increased cognitive reserve

"Cognitive reserve" refers to how flexibly and efficiently we utilize our brain reserve, which includes brain size and neuronal count[4]. Education, work, and other activities related to *Keep Learning* protect the brain and help us compensate for declines in certain brain functions. Those of us with greater cognitive reserve can accomplish more mentally at any given level of brain pathology. Cognitive reserve predicts higher cognitive and functional outcomes following brain injury, as well as reduced cognitive decline over time. People with greater cognitive reserve have greater reductions in both brain cortical thickness and regional atrophy before symptoms of Alzheimer's disease appear[4]. Thus, greater cognitive reserve appears to compensate for Alzheimer's-type brain pathologies.

Reduced risk of dementia and cognitive decline

Dementia isn't a specific disease; it's a chronic disorder of mental processes arising from injury or illness. The symptoms include impaired memory, defective reasoning, or altered personality. Alzheimer's-type dementia accounts for 60–80 percent of all dementia cases. Alzheimer's, in which brain cells die and connections between cells are lost, affects between four and five million Americans each year, and exacts an annual monetary cost of roughly $226 billion[5]. Current drug treatments may lessen symptoms for a limited time but are unable to stem the damage the disease causes to brain cells. Thus, adopting healthy lifestyle choices may be the best way to reduce the risk of dementia and prevent or slow the rate of cognitive decline with advancing age.

Mild cognitive impairment: mental deterioration that lies below that of normal cognitive function as identified by individuals, family members, or clinicians, but without significant impairment in daily activities.

Clinical Alzheimer's-type dementia: cognitive impairment severe enough that an individual can no longer function independently[6].

A meta-analysis of 22 studies found that, compared to persons with low levels of mental activity, those with high levels had a 36 percent lower risk of dementia. Having more education, greater occupational complexity, and greater cognitive lifestyle activities predicted comparable reductions in dementia risk. Several mechanisms might explain why mental activity protects against dementia. Mental stimulation induces the production of neurotrophins, chemicals that support the growth and survival of neurons and which are linked to mental acuity. Mental activity promotes synaptic plasticity, creates new synapses between nerve cells, and promotes nerve cell production in the hippocampus, the part of the brain that plays a critical role in memory[7].

Several studies link mentally stimulating activities of older people to a lower risk of mental deterioration. The Rush Memory and Aging Project in Chicago collected data annually for up to five years from elderly participants (mean age of 80 years) regarding cognitive function and cognitive disorders. Researchers found that subjects who reported more frequent engagement in cognitive activities (such as reading a newspaper, playing chess, visiting a library) had a lower risk of Alzheimer's disease. More specifically, participants in the top ten percent of cognitive activity had a 42 percent lower risk of developing Alzheimer's disease compared to participants in the bottom ten

Three Combined Actions May Reduce Risk for Alzheimer's

A new report from the National Academy of Sciences addressed the issue of preventing cognitive decline and dementia[10]. Encouraging evidence suggests that combining: (1) cognitive training, (2) blood pressure management for people with hypertension, and (3) increased physical activity may reduce the risk of clinical Alzheimer's-type dementia. The experts cautioned, however, that existing evidence does not support creating a public health campaign to promote these three actions for dementia prevention. Nevertheless, cognitive training, reducing blood pressure to safe levels, and increasing physical activity all promote other aspects of health and well-being. So even if these three healthy choices don't reduce the risk of Alzheimer's disease or mild cognitive impairment, they're still worth doing.

percent of cognitive activity. More frequent cognitive activities also predicted a lower risk of mild cognitive impairment and less rapid cognitive decline. Increased cognitive activity earlier in life might build a cognitive reserve that could reduce the risk of developing Alzheimer's disease and counter the adverse effects of brain pathologies[8]. Further trials are needed to provide conclusive evidence of the cause and effect of specific techniques to prevent or ameliorate dementia[9]. In the meantime, why not live on the safe side and *Keep Learning*?

Increased goal-directed activity

We've all had the experience of doing something and then recognizing an opportunity to make progress toward an unrelated goal that we'd pushed to the back burner. Here's an explanation of how this works, according to researchers Colleen Seifert and Andrea Patalano[11]:

1. We put a goal on the mental back burner because it doesn't fit with our current priorities.

2. We consider the required circumstances for the goal's completion.

3. We "encode" the postponed goal into memory associated with the circumstances for the goal's completion.

4. The associated circumstances appear in our life.

5. When we perceive the associated circumstances, we bring the goal to mind.

6. We decide whether or not to resume working on the goal.

Keep Learning might help us remember back-burner goals and act on them when appropriate occasions arise.

Development of new life skills

In his book *Creating Significant Learning Opportunities*, L. Dee Fink[12] argues that learning is an integral part of the dance of life. In the past, many adults felt that they didn't need to learn much in formal and informal settings, especially beyond high school. That has changed. These days, adults must continue to learn in order to develop new salable skills and acquire knowledge to prepare for future jobs, which may have not yet been invented. Fink distinguishes between individual intentional learning and formal learning programs. Individual intentional learning refers to projects that adults under-take on their own for self-improvement, such as reading a self-help book like this one, or learning a new techno-skill. Formal learning programs include those organized by a specific person or organization and made available to the general public. For example, many universities, colleges, and public school districts offer online classes. Fink advises us to see ourselves as proactive, self-directed, lifelong learners, because that mindset will expand our horizons, improve our health and well-being, and change us as people. Seeing ourselves as lifelong learners can help us *Keep Learning* as long as we live.

Improved balance

Older people often experience diminished balance. This reduces *Quality of Lifespan* by making walking more difficult and increasing the risk of falls and fractures. Hip fracture in older people is a leading cause of admission to nursing homes. Balance skills have been associated with the hippocampus, a small area of the brain involved not only in memory but also in spatial cognition and motor skills. Although the hippocampus atrophies with age, it can generate new neurons throughout life.

Because dancing combines aerobic fitness, sensorimotor skills, and cognitive demands, researchers wanted to know if dancing could improve balance in older people and possibly reduce the risk of injury. Sixty-two subjects with an average age of 67 were randomized into either dancing or sports training groups. Both groups met for 90 minutes twice a week for six months, then once a week for 90 minutes for 12 months. The dancing group performed a variety of moves in various dance forms, while the sports group performed endurance, strength, and flexibility training. Hippocampal volume was determined at baseline, six, and 12 months from magnetic resonance images. While both groups showed increased volume in the left hippocampus, only the dance group significantly increased the volume in two other specific portions of the hippocampus (left dentate gyrus, right subiculum). This study showed that both dancing and fitness training can induce hippocampal plasticity, but only dancing improved balance[13].

Improved growth mindset

Carol Dweck at Stanford University developed the concept of fixed and growth mindsets. People with a fixed mindset tend to regard their intelligence as formed at birth and impervious to improvement. Such people tend to think that their successes reflect their innate intelligence, and that their failures reveal limits to their intelligence. On the other hand, people with a growth mindset tend to regard intelligence as malleable, and that their successes reflect effort as much as or more than intelligence. Growth mindset people tend to regard failure as reflecting a poor application of effort.

Given the above, wouldn't it be wonderful if a growth mindset could be taught? In fact, Dweck and her colleagues demonstrated that adolescents could learn a growth mindset, which resulted in improved academic performance in middle school. The study sought to determine if students' beliefs about their intelligence would predict mathematics performance. The study involved weekly 25-minute sessions with experimental and control groups over eight weeks and tracked 373 middle school students over two years. Sessions 1, 2, 5, and 6 (dealing with the structure and function of the brain; an anti-stereotyping lesson) were identical in both groups, while sessions 3, 4, 7, and 8 differed. In the latter sessions, students in the experimental group read aloud in class about the growth mindset and discussed how learning could make them smarter. Students in the control group read aloud about memory and discussed academic difficulties and successes. At the beginning of the study, students with fixed and growth mindsets showed no differences in math scores. However, over the two years of the study, the math scores of students with a growth mindset exceeded the scores of students with a fixed mindset. Students who believed that intelligence was malleable pursued their learning goals more diligently and were more likely to believe that working hard was necessary for learning than those who thought

Learn That Intelligence is Malleable

Could a brief, one-time intervention change students' views of the malleability of their personality, leading to more resourceful responses toward adverse events in life? The answer is yes! A single 25-minute intervention used reading and writing to teach the growth mindset of personality: Socially relevant aspects can be changed. Three groups of students entering high school who received the intervention self-reported reduced depressive symptoms nine months afterward, compared to control groups that did not receive the intervention. This and similar studies indicate that brief interventions have the potential to induce positive, long-term behavioral changes that can motivate us to adopt better choices and improve our overall health and well-being[16].

intelligence was fixed. Students with a growth mindset were less likely to make ability-based attributions and feel helpless when faced with a challenging situation compared to students with a fixed mindset[14].

Practical Ways to *Keep Learning*

The following actions will help you *Keep Learning*. The most effective ones may be activities that are novel for you. Especially useful are those that involve either moving your body in space or using hand-eye coordination. Dancing, table tennis, and learning to play a musical instrument fit the bill nicely.

- **Dance.** Dancing helps maintain and build neural connections. If dancing is new to you, the rewards can be especially great. Most communities offer opportunities for social dancing or dance lessons. Why not give it a try?

- **Adopt a growth mindset.** Interventions that foster a growth mindset have profound implications. First, they show that our thoughts and beliefs affect how we learn. Second, if we adopt a growth mindset, we'll be more likely to adopt the healthy choice of lifelong learning and more likely will enjoy greater success in the world. People with a growth mindset are far more likely to *Keep Learning* and thrive in tomorrow's world than those with a fixed mindset. Read Carol Dweck's book *Mindset* for more information[15].

- **Train your brain.** Research demonstrates that the human brain is far more plastic than previously realized. Training the brain can improve certain aspects of cognitive function, such as memory enhancement[17].

- **Create and maintain active intellectual and social engagement.** Active social engagement fosters learning and predicts lower risk of developing dementia. Based on longitudinal studies, leisure activities that most strongly predict a reduced risk of dementia include reading, visiting friends or relatives, going to movies or restaurants, and walking for pleasure or on an excursion[18]. Maintaining intellectual and social engagement through participation in everyday activities seems to buffer healthy individuals against cognitive decline in later life, possibly by creating cognitive reserve.

- **Practice mindfulness meditation.** Mindfulness meditation might help build cognitive reserve directly, through repeated activations of attention focusing, and indirectly through improved stress reduction and immune function. Recent research suggests that mindfulness meditation improves a range of cognitive functions, including sustained attention, attention control, and working memory. Mindfulness meditation might improve brain networks involved in specific cognitive functions, or boost brain states that control a range of neural networks affecting many cognitive processes. Research also suggests that meditation improves neural network efficiency for tasks far removed from those practiced in meditation[19].

Three Key Points

1. The brain is far more malleable than previously thought, even in older people.

2. Learning new skills (such as dancing) that integrate body and mind can help build cognitive reserve, which can offset the negative effects of brain pathologies.

3. Becoming an enthusiastic lifelong learner can increase our engagement with life and may reduce our risk of cognitive problems in later years.

Part 3

Nurture Your Spirit with Three Healthy Choices

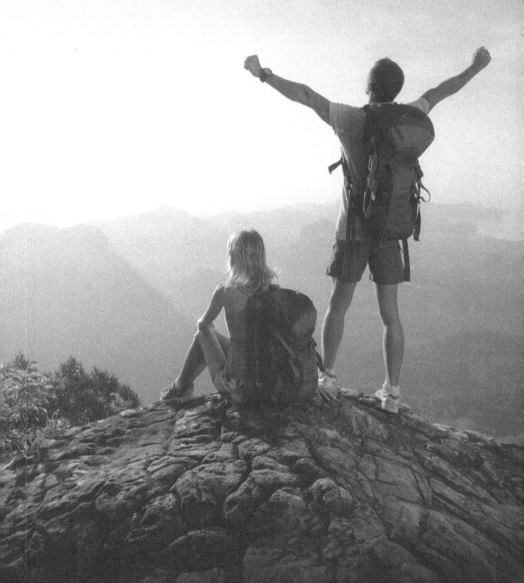

Chapter 7

Develop a Positive
Mental Attitude

Choose to be optimistic, it feels better.
— Dalai Lama XIV

The concept of a positive mental attitude has its popular origins in the writing of Napoleon Hill[1]. His classic book, *Think and Grow Rich*, first published in 1937, emphasized the importance of positive thinking as a key ingredient in a successful life. The phrase "positive mental attitude" appeared in the title of one his of later books, *Success Through a Positive Mental Attitude*, which he co-authored with W. Clement Stone. The fact that our mind exerts a profound impact on our health and well-being supports the healthy choice of *Develop a Positive Mental Attitude*.

This chapter highlights optimism, gratitude, and forgiveness, three important attributes of a positive mental attitude that can help us achieve lifelong vibrant health and emotional well-being.

The Power of Positive Expectations

Would you believe we can imagine our way to better health? That may sound crazy, but it's true—our brain can convince our body to respond positively to a sham intervention simply because we anticipate that it will help us. This beneficial medical outcome, based on our positive expectation of it, is called the placebo effect. In fact, 60–90 percent of drugs and other therapies prescribed by physicians depend on the placebo effect for their effectiveness. Curiously, research supports the hypothesis that exercise improves health, in part, through the placebo effect. More on that later.

Placebo effect

Within the scientific community, there is no doubt that the placebo effect exists. Psychologist Alan Roberts analyzed 27 studies of five different medical procedures performed by physicians who all believed in the procedures' effectiveness, and who told their patients that these various approaches were promising. Of the 6,913 patients receiving one or more procedures—*all later found to be ineffective*—40 percent reported excellent results, 21 percent reported good results, and 30 percent reported poor results. Roberts concluded that both the subjects and the doctors held hopeful expectations regarding these procedures. The predominance of reported "excellent" results of procedures later deemed ineffective suggested that the heightened expectation for a successful outcome accounted for a sizeable proportion of reported positive outcomes. This study supports the proposition that *our mind creates the life we experience,* even if we aren't consciously aware of it[2].

To test the hypothesis that exercise affects health partially through the placebo effect, one study tracked 84 cleaning attendants at seven hotels. Typical work tasks involved walking, bending, lifting and shoving furniture, and carrying trash bags—clearly meeting the U.S. Surgeon General's recommended minimum of 30 minutes of daily moderate-intensity exercise. Forty-four subjects in the "informed" group were told that their work activity was good exercise and that it met the recommended minimum level of daily exercise. Forty subjects in the "uninformed" group were not told this. All the subjects were told about the general benefits of exercise. Baseline health measures indicated that the subjects' perception of their health was worse than it actually was and that they were unaware of the health benefits of their work. After one month, subjects in the informed group showed a significant increase in their perception of their work as exercise, compared to the uninformed subjects. Furthermore, the informed subjects had improved measures of health—body weight, body-mass index, percentage of body fat, waist-hip ratio, and blood pressure—compared to the uninformed subjects. Thus, simply perceiving work as exercise may lead to improved physiological health[3].

Can our beliefs about our abilities and expectations for the future affect our performance? Those of us who've played competitive sports will say yes. A recent study provides support. Thirty-one university students were assigned to either the heightened-expectancy group or the control group. Both groups had to throw a tennis ball 20 times (overhand in baseball fashion) at a target seven meters (23 feet) away, striking the target as close to

Beliefs and Expectations Influence Placebo Effect

The ethical rub regarding studies of the placebo effect is that research subjects are essentially misled into thinking the pills they take or the procedure they undergo will improve their health. But what would happen if the placebo in a clinical trial were advertised as such?

Researchers tested this question. Eighty mostly female subjects with irritable bowel syndrome were assigned to one of two groups.

Subjects in the placebo group received pills openly labeled as inert or inactive (with no medication), but they were told that the pills had been shown in rigorous clinical trials to produce significant mind-body healing.

Subjects in the no treatment group did not receive any placebo pills, but they did receive the same amount and type of patient-provider contact as those in the placebo group.

Patients in the placebo group had significantly better scores on four measures of irritable bowel syndrome, both at the study's midpoint (day 11) and at the study's end (day 21).

the center as possible. After completing the throws, participants assessed their overall sense of volition and self-determination by answering two questionnaires. All participants were informed that the questionnaires would be used to create a performance index (PI) to predict performance under pressure.

The positive result of the placebo may have arisen from participants believing in the value of the placebo effect in spite of being informed that the placebo contained no medication. Beliefs and expectations can be powerful forces to improve health[4].

Participants in the heightened-expectancy group were told that low PI scores predicted who would do poorly in the next round of throws and that high PI scores predicted who would do well. Next, all the high-expectancy participants were told that they received very high scores. Control participants were told that the questionnaires were used to determine their PI and that the study was designed to evaluate how scores related to performance under pressure. Participants in both groups were informed that they would win a prize if they and a randomly selected partner would both improve their scores by 15 percent or more.

Participants in both groups completed a second round of 20 throws and then responded to a final set of questions about their ability to perform under pressure. Members of the heightened-expectancy group improved their accuracy scores from the first (low-pressure) round of throws to the second (high-pressure) round, while the control group stayed nearly the same. Participants in the heightened-expectancy group were more likely to reach the 15 percent improvement goal than those in the control group. Telling participants that they were likely to do well under pressure resulted in greater perceived ability. A heightened expectancy increased their throwing accuracy[5]. The bottom line: If we can convince ourselves that we're competent in the game of life, we're more likely to do better.

Perceived Sense of Control and Self-Efficacy

Sadly, many older people hold negative stereotypes of aging, such as the belief that age-related declines are undesirable, inevitable, and irreversible. While genetic factors do influence aging, beliefs about control and self-confidence figure prominently in how we age. People with a positive mental attitude are likely to feel they have a measure of control over their lives and are more likely to have positive emotions. Research suggests that a perceived sense of control over one's life promotes better health and well-being. For example, greater perceived control is linked with fewer chronic conditions, less depression, fewer functional limitations, better memory, reduced stress response, and faster recovery from illness. What a list!

Perceived control is also associated with an increased socioeconomic status and education level. Perhaps people who experience success in the world over time develop a sense of control. This sense of control can influence feelings of self-efficacy (self-confidence), competence, and positive expectations about the future. A sense of control typically declines in late adulthood, but perceived control can be learned; diminished perceived control is not inevitable in old age. Maintaining a sense of control late in life may occur in areas we deem especially important. For example, we may want to maintain control over our physical function so we can play with our grandkids. Research suggests that older people who develop a greater sense of control over their lives can enjoy better health and well-being[6].

Psychologist Albert Bandura wrote extensively about self-efficacy, namely, persons' beliefs that they are capable of performing a particular behavior. High self-efficacy fosters a "can-do" attitude. Bandura proposed that high self-efficacy is the number one component of developing motivation to engage in healthy behaviors. In other words, people who believe they are capable of performing actions that will improve their health are more likely to engage in them, especially over the long term, compared to people who believe they're incapable.

How, then, can we increase our self-efficacy? According to Bandura, a can-do attitude can be fostered in several ways: by developing mastery; through vicarious experiences of others with whom we can identify; with social persuasion via verbal encouragement in our ability to succeed; by creating situations in which we are likely to succeed; and by reducing our stress reactions and altering our interpretations of stress[7].

Self-Efficacy Promotes Healthy Behaviors in Cardiac Patients

British researchers used data from patients at two hospitals in southern England to learn whether patients with coronary heart disease who exhibited greater self-efficacy would be more likely to undertake healthy behaviors than patients with lower self-efficacy. Between baseline and three years later, patients who went through an individualized cardiac rehab program increased their confidence in the ability to exercise more, while patients in a generic cardiac rehab program did not. Promoting patients' management of their perceived symptoms, increasing their self-efficacy, increasing their sense of control over their illness, and helping them realize that cardiac illness is a long-term condition appeared to promote long-term exercise habits. The initial belief that the patients' cardiac conditions were controllable predicted their ability to continue exercising over the three-year period of the study[8].

Positive and Negative Perceptions of Aging

Negative perceptions of aging can profoundly affect our health. Fortunately, we can change these perceptions. In so doing, we can greatly increase our likelihood of aging successfully. Figure 7.1 summarizes ways in which positive self-perceptions of aging can lead to improved health outcomes.

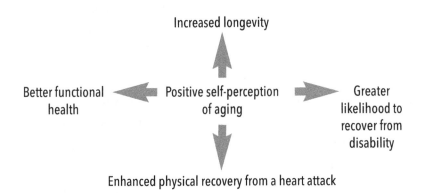

Figure 7.1. Positive perceptions of aging can lead to positive health outcomes.

Ralph Waldo Emerson wrote, "You become what you think about all day long." If Emerson was correct, it follows that our self-perceptions of aging affect how we age. If we expect that aging will be negative (infirmity, illness, loss of independence), it will probably turn out that way. On the other hand, if we expect that aging will be positive (greater wisdom, time to reflect upon our life, greater patience), it has every chance of becoming just that.

Australian researchers used data from a longitudinal study of aging to understand how self-perceptions of aging manifested in later life. The study included a representative sample of Australian residents at least 70 years old, starting in 1992–1993 and ending in 2007–2008. Participants who developed positive self-perceptions of aging earlier in life lived longer than those who didn't develop early, positive self-perceptions of aging. We can infer from these findings that people with positive self-perceptions of aging might be more likely to adopt healthy habits or to follow doctors' advice, thereby leading to longer life[9].

Optimism

The field of positive psychology seeks to understand what makes life worth living. The field's premier researcher, Martin Seligman, and his colleagues have amassed overwhelming evidence that people with an optimistic outlook live better than pessimists[10]. Optimists are healthier, live longer, make more money, and are happier than pessimists. Seligman even demonstrated that professional athletic teams that have an optimistic outlook outperform teams with a negative outlook.

Optimism is associated with a variety of positive mental and physical health factors (Figure 7.2). However, optimism is just one of several attributes within the broader concept of psychological well-being. Cardiologist Alan Rozanski urges reframing optimism into the broader perspective of enhancing psychological well-being and vitality, which can occur through several pathways. Rozanski proposes developing cost-effective integrated programs that provide support and counseling across a range of disciplines, including exercise, nutrition, sleep hygiene, and behavior. Such programs could reduce the prevalence of risk factors, such as sedentary living, poor diet, and insufficient sleep, all of which can be reversed by making better choices[11].

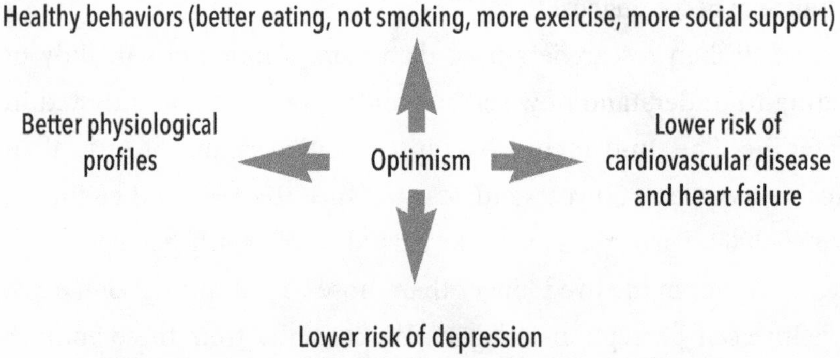

Healthy behaviors (better eating, not smoking, more exercise, more social support)

Better physiological profiles ← Optimism → Lower risk of cardiovascular disease and heart failure

Lower risk of depression

Figure 7.2. Potential health and well-being benefits of optimism.

Optimism has been conceptualized in two different ways. The *explanatory style* centers on the notion that bad events are temporary, limited, and impersonal rather than ongoing, broadly applicable, and persona. *Dispositional optimism* refers to the general belief that good things rather than bad things will happen. Dispositional optimism has been associated with a variety of positive health behaviors, biological processes, and cardiovascular outcomes. For instance, optimistic people are more likely to engage in behaviors that reduce the risk of cardiovascular disease, such as not smoking, exercising regularly, and eating better.

Gratitude

According to Robert Emmons in his book *Thanks!: How the New Science of Gratitude Can Make You Happier*, gratitude means acknowledging the goodness in our own life and recognizing that the source of goodness lies partially outside of ourselves[12]. If we regularly practice gratitude, we'll likely reap a host of emotional, physical, and personal benefits. Emmons, a pioneer in the psychology of gratitude, writes that feeling grateful creates a ripple effect through all aspects of our lives, including our quest for inner peace, wholeness, and contentment.

Forgiveness

Fred Luskin co-founded and directs the Stanford University Forgiveness Project. His book *Forgive for Good* provides a readable and helpful account of how we can use forgiveness to get over long-term grievances that sap positive energy in our lives[13]. According to Luskin, forgiveness has several key characteristics, including taking responsibility for how we feel, taking back our power, getting control over our feelings, and improving our mental and physical heath. Forgiveness is a choice that we can make. Happily, forgiveness is learnable just like any other skill. Bad things may happen to us, but that does not mean that we have to dwell on them. It's also important to remember that dwelling on the past won't change it. But we can change how we regard the past and act appropriately in the present.

Happiness

In her book *The How of Happiness – A New Approach to Getting the Life You Want*, researcher Sonja Lyubomirksy defines happiness as "the experience of joy, contentment, or positive well-being combined with a sense that one's life is good, meaningful, and worthwhile." By this definition, studies show that happy people have more energy, creativity, higher immune system function, higher income, better mental health, and greater longevity than people who aren't happy[14]. One study of Catholic nuns, who were observed over 60 years, revealed a seven-year gain in longevity between the most and least happy nuns[15]. Other research showed that a person's happiness is 15 percent greater when he or she is connected to another happy person.

Positivity

Positivity is the quality of being encouraging or promising a successful outcome. Numerous experiments conducted by the most influential researcher on the subject, Barbara Fredrickson, and others demonstrate that people with high positivity scores are more optimistic, more resilient, more open, more accepting, and more driven by purpose than people with low positivity scores. If that isn't enough, a meta-analysis of 300 published studies revealed that positivity was correlated with greater success in life, a satisfying marriage, a larger salary, and better health[16].

Benefits Linked to *Develop a Positive Mental Attitude*

We all know people who view the glass as half full and others who see it as half empty. While it's true that our personality influences our attitude, and life circumstances can certainly affect it as well, those things don't necessarily have to determine our attitude. If we learn to *Develop a Positive Mental Attitude* toward life, we may experience many benefits.

Benefits Linked to *Develop a Positive Mental Attitude*

- Increased longevity
- Reduced risk of premature death
- Reduced risk of cardiovascular disease
- Reduced risk of hospitalization
- Improved overall health
- Improved functional health
- Increased likelihood of making healthy choices
- Increased well-being
- Greater use of preventive health services
- Reduced risk of cognitive impairment
- Faster recovery from disability
- Healthy aging

Increased longevity

Part of developing a positive mental attitude involves developing positive thoughts and beliefs about growing older. However, American cultural norms do not often support positive thoughts and beliefs about aging. In 2002, researchers examined data from an earlier study to determine whether negative perceptions toward aging could affect longevity. Researchers previously contacted nearly all residents of Oxford, Ohio, who were cognitively intact and at least 50 years of age. Five hundred and sixty people between ages 50 and 94 were followed for an average of 23 years. This study found that participants with a high positive self-perception of aging lived an average of 7.5 years longer than participants with a low positive self-perception of aging. An astounding difference! Attitude had a greater effect on longevity than did reducing blood pressure or cholesterol[17]. If a big pharmaceutical company developed a pill that would increase longevity by 7.5 years with no side effects, it would make a fortune. But we don't need a pill, do we?

Reduced risk of premature death

According to researchers Corey Keyes and Eduardo Simoes, people with overall subjective well-being have emotional well-being (feeling good) and social and psychological well-being (functioning well-being). Flourishing reflects the combination of emotional, social, and psychological well-being. Keyes and Simoes used data from 2,440 participants ranging in age from 25 to 74 at baseline in the MIDUS cohort study to determine if flourishing predicted mortality. Results showed that non-flourishing adults had a 62 percent higher risk of dying over the ten-year follow-up period than the flourishing adults, after accounting for a host of confounding factors. Less than 1 percent of adults flourishing at baseline died during the ten-year follow-up period, compared to 5.5 percent of the non-flourishing adults[18].

Dispositional optimism—the belief that good rather than bad things will generally happen—predicts better health and a lower risk of mortality. Dutch researchers sought to determine if this applied to older people. Participants in the Arnhem Elderly Study, which began in 1991–1992, served as the research subjects. After an average of 9.1 years, researchers found that, compared with subjects with a high level of pessimism, subjects reporting a high level of optimism had a 45 percent lower risk of all-cause mortality. When the risk was adjusted for potentially confounding factors such as age, education, and smoking, the all-cause risk of dying for subjects reporting high levels of optimism shrank to 15 percent. For cardiovascular mortality, the risk for subjects with high levels of optimism was 14 or 19 percent, depending on which potentially confounding factors appeared in the statistical model. Regardless of sociodemographic and cardiovascular risk factors, dispositional optimism predicted lower all-cause mortality and cardiovascular mortality in older people[19].

Heart failure is a leading cause of death in the U.S. Researchers used data from the Health and Retirement study starting in 1992 that recruited samples of Americans over age 50. The study included 6,808 participants (at least 65 years old, with a mean age of 70 at baseline). After four years, each standard deviation increase in optimism scores was associated with a 26 percent lower rate of developing heart failure. When optimism scores were grouped in quartiles from lowest to highest, the rate of heart failure decreased in a dose-response relationship, indicating a cause-and-effect relationship. Compared with participants in the lowest quartile of optimism scores, participants in the low-moderate, moderate-high, and high quartiles had a 25, 31, and 48 percent lower rates of hospitalization, respectively[20]. If we increase our level of optimism, we may substantially reduce our risk of heart failure and hospitalization.

A study investigated the link between depression and cardiovascular disease mortality in 11,263 middle-aged men who were initially free of, but at high risk for, coronary heart disease, a form of cardiovascular disease. Participants were followed for an average of 18 years after being evaluated for depressive symptoms using a standard 20-item questionnaire. Compared to participants who reported no depressive symptoms at baseline, those in the highest quintile of depressive symptoms had double the risk of cardiovascular disease mortality (mostly due to stroke). As depressive symptoms increased, the risk of death from stroke increased in a dose-response manner, suggesting cause-and-effect. Thus, developing a positive mental attitude may reduce our risk of depression and also reduce the risk of stroke and other cardiovascular diseases[21].

Greater optimism predicts lower risk of all-cause mortality and mortality from cardiovascular disease. But what about other chronic conditions? Do optimistic people enjoy a lower risk of death from causes such as stroke, respiratory disease, infection, and cancer? Researchers addressed this question using data from 70,021 women who participated in the Nurses' Health Study. Scientists found that serum cholesterol, hypertension, type 2 diabetes, and depression declined in a graded manner as optimism scores increased. Compared to participants in the lowest quartile of optimism, participants in the highest quartile had a significantly lower risk of all-cause mortality. Similarly, compared to those in the lowest quartile of optimism, those in the highest quartile had a significantly lower risk of dying from heart disease, stroke, respiratory disease, infection, and all-cause cancer. The reductions in risk for nurses in the most optimistic quartile were 38, 39, 37, 52, and 16 percent for heart disease, stroke, respiratory disease, infection, and total cancer, respectively, compared to nurses in the lowest quartile. This study was one of the first to demonstrate significant associations between optimism and broad measures of health in a general U.S. population sample. Given that optimism can be learned, interventions that promote optimism may improve health by preventing chronic diseases[22].

Two British researchers conducted meta-analyses of studies that investigated mortality in initially healthy and diseased populations, respectively. The protective effects of positive psychological well-being occurred independently of negative affect (bad mood). Positive psychological well-being was associated with reduced all-cause mortality in both healthy and diseased populations. Additionally, positive psychological well-being in healthy populations was significantly associated with reduced cardiovascular mortality. Aspects of both positive affect (such as emotional well-being, positive mood, joy, happiness, vigor, energy) and positive trait-like dispositions (such as life satisfaction, hopefulness, optimism, sense of humor) were associated with reduced mortality in healthy populations[23].

Reduced risk of cardiovascular disease

Recent research shows that positive affect contributes not only to increased survival, better immune function, and lower risk of certain chronic conditions, but also lowers the risk of a particular form of cardiovascular disease, namely coronary heart disease. Researchers used data on 1,739 Canadian adults with no recent history of cardiovascular disease and who were followed for ten years. The risk of coronary heart disease declined in a linear manner as the subjects' positive affect scores increased from one to five. Subjects with a high positive affect score of five had a 62 percent lower risk of coronary heart disease compared to subjects with a low positive affect score of one. The dose-response relationship suggests that greater positive affect caused reduced risk of coronary heart disease [24].

In another study, researchers from Harvard University reviewed the association between positive psychological well-being and cardiovascular disease. Psychological well-being included purpose/meaning in life, transient feelings of life satisfaction, and optimism. The review revealed that positive psychological well-being consistently protected against cardiovascular disease, regardless of traditional risk factors and health status. Optimism, followed by transient feelings of life satisfaction and a sense of purpose/meaning in life, was most robustly associated with reduced risk of cardiovascular events. Positive psychological well-being was positively associated with restorative health behaviors and biological function and inversely associated with deteriorative health behaviors and biological function[25]. The takeaway message: People with an optimistic outlook on life, and to a lesser extent people with high life satisfaction and purpose in life, are likely to enjoy better cardiovascular health than pessimistic people.

Several studies show a relationship between hostility and aspects of cardiovascular disease in older adults. Also, hostility earlier in life predicts coronary artery calcification in young adults. Coronary artery calcification occurs early in the process of coronary artery plaque development, which can lead to cardiovascular disease. In 387 young adults, aged 18–30, coronary artery calcification was measured at ten years post-baseline. Compared with participants who scored below the median on global hostility, those who scored above the median (the more hostile participants) had a 157 percent higher risk of coronary artery calcification, after accounting for potentially confounding factors. Thus, it appears that young adults who reduce their global hostility may reduce their risk of cardiovascular disease[26].

Positivity Lowers Risk for a Second Heart Attack

Researchers interviewed 287 heart attack patients seven weeks and again eight years after their heart attack. Patients who cited benefits from their misfortune—presumably reflecting greater optimism—seven weeks after the first attack were less likely to have another attack and had lower levels of cardiovascular illness eight years later. Attributing the initial attack to stress responses (such as worrying or nervousness) predicted greater illness in eight-year survivors. Blaming the initial attack on other people predicted a follow-up heart attack. Men who survived a subsequent heart attack were more likely than men who did not have additional attacks to cite benefits and lack of earlier positive health habits eight years after the initial attack[27].

Reduced risk of hospitalization

People with positive self-perceptions of aging are more likely to attribute age-related bodily changes to modifiable factors (such as insufficient exercise) and make healthier choices than those with a negative self-perception. To test whether older people who make more frequent healthy choices would have fewer overnight hospitalizations, researchers examined data from 4,735 participants (mean age 69 years at baseline) in the Health and Retirement Study. When scores were grouped in quartiles from lower (worse) self-perceptions of aging to higher (better) self-perceptions of aging, the rate of hospitalizations decreased sequentially, indicating a dose-response relationship[28]. Compared with participants in the lowest, most negative, quartile of self-perception of aging scores, participants in the low-moderate, moderate-high, and high quartiles had 33, 36, and 55 percent lower rates of hospitalization, respectively. If we can minimize our in-patient hospital visits, just think how much we can help reduce medical costs as the U.S. population ages and help limit health insurance cost increases.

Generally speaking, positive psychological factors appear to support positive health outcomes. But a recent study showed that optimism, rather than gratitude, predicted a significantly greater level of physical activity (measured as step counts) 6.5 months after a diagnosis of acute cardiac syndrome. Similarly, optimism significantly predicted fewer hospital cardiac readmissions at 6.5 months. Optimism, being a forward-looking concept, may align better with the forward-looking process of recovery from cardiac ailments, while gratitude focuses more on the present. In addition, optimism may work its magic indirectly by promoting healthy lifestyle choices, rather than operating directly on the body's physiology[29].

Improved overall health

A doctoral dissertation from the University of Wisconsin examined the relationship between forgiveness of interpersonal hurts and self-reported physical health. After controlling for a variety of demographic and health-risk factors, forgiveness and the number of recent or chronic health symptoms were significantly negatively correlated. Likewise, forgiveness was significantly negatively correlated with the number of medically diagnosed chronic health conditions and the prevalence of hypertension and heart disease. In other words, the study's findings suggest that forgiving serious interpersonal injuries predicts better physical health. Finally, hostility—a near-opposite of forgiveness—significantly predicted negative health outcomes. Interestingly, the failure to forgive was a better predictor of physical health problems than was hostility[30].

Considerable longitudinal research links optimism with various measures of better health and well-being, including reduced mortality risk, better self-reported health, fewer sick days, slower transition from HIV infection to AIDS, better measures of aging, reduced pain, reduced effects of falling, and reduced risk of stroke. Evidently, optimists tend to make more healthy choices than pessimists. Studies suggest that optimists are healthier than pessimists because optimists act differently than pessimists, in line with positive perceptions and expectations. A study of identical twins found that only 25 percent of optimism arises from one's genes. Optimism can be learned. Less clear is whether interventions designed to enhance optimism cause better health. Even if they don't, research shows that optimism enhances lifelong well-being with no or minimal side effects[31].

Salubrious effects of optimism might arise directly from the neuroendocrine system and from immune responses. Alternatively, the effects might appear indirectly by promoting positive health behaviors, improving coping strategies, and fostering a positive mood. The benefits of optimism come from what might be called realistic optimism: anticipating positive outcomes in the future, tempered by practical considerations. Most studies focus on dispositional optimism, which is considered to be a character trait. Dispositional optimism, however, can be learned. Optimists tend to view desired goals, such as improving health, as attainable. Thus, they tend to approach adversities actively, thereby increasing their odds of goal attainment. Dispositional optimism predicts psychological well-being, positive mood, perseverance, and effective problem solving, better health, and longer life. Optimism is strongly associated with improved emotional and behavioral adjustment to cancer diagnosis, perhaps by helping patients find meaning in the experience. Overall, optimism is significantly linked to various measures of positive health[32].

To understand whether optimism changes with age in older adults and, if so, how that might affect health, researchers used data from 9,790 older adults who were part of the Health and Retirement Study. Participants in the 2006 and 2012 groups were followed for up to four years. Researchers found that optimism increased until age 68 but declined thereafter. However, increases in optimism over the four-year period between baseline and follow-up were associated with improvements in self-reported health[33]. Thus, learning how to be more optimistic might help seniors live healthier.

The experience of a heart attack can motivate people to make major lifestyle changes. A British study followed 143 first-time heart attack patients, mostly middle-aged men, for six month after hospital admission. Beliefs of the patients and of their spouses significantly predicted post-heart attack behaviors. The patients most strongly attributed their heart attack to stress, high cholesterol, and eating fatty foods, while their spouses cited stress, high cholesterol, and heredity. Patients who attributed their heart attack to lifestyle causes showed significant improvements in diet and exercise. Spousal attribution of a heart attack to a lifestyle cause predicted significantly more exercise of the patient. If we believe that our health problems arise from poor lifestyle choices, we may be more motivated to make better lifestyle choices in the future[34].

Improved functional health

Functional health refers to the ability to perform normal activities of daily living, such as bathing, toileting, and eating. Researchers used data from 433 participants in the Ohio Longitudinal Study of Aging and Retirement who enrolled in 1975 with a median follow-up of 22.6 years. Subjects with more positive self-perceptions of aging at baseline were significantly more likely to have better functional health over the ensuing years. Moreover, the difference of functional health between subjects with positive self-perceptions of aging and those with negative self-perceptions increased over time[17].

Making healthy choices can truly help us create lifelong vibrant health and emotional well-being. Researchers used data from 4,238 subjects enrolled in the Midlife in the United States study (1995–1966 and 2002–2006) to investigate the relationship between combined psychosocial and behavioral factors and functional limitations. The protective factors the researchers considered included control beliefs, quality of social support, and exercise. Higher control beliefs, better social support, and more exercise (individually and collectively) predicted maintaining functional health from baseline to ten years later. Functional health of older subjects with the three protective factors was greater than that for middle-aged subjects with one or no protective factors[35]. If we *Develop a Positive Mental Attitude, Cultivate Social Support,* and *Keep Moving,* we're more likely to maintain functionality into old age and improve our *Quality of Lifespan.*

Increased likelihood of making healthy choices

Finding ways to encourage older Americans to engage in health-promoting behaviors could lead to reduced health care costs. Not surprisingly, several aspects of motivation play an important role in positive health behavior. The famous Terman Study, which began in 1921 and followed 1,500 gifted fifth graders for the rest of their lives, sheds light on this. Around the year 2000, a questionnaire was mailed to 298 surviving participants of the study; completed questionnaires were received from 162 respondents. Positive health behavior was evaluated using the following: (1) exercising and being physically active, (2) getting enough sleep, (3) getting enough relaxation, (4) eating well, (5) controlling weight, (6)

Positive Thinking and Recovering from Surgery

On November 1, 2016, my wife Betsy had her left hip replaced. Prior to the operation, she developed the mindset that her operation would be a complete success. Betsy did her homework checking out surgeons in the Denver metro area. She wanted to have total confidence that her surgeon was the best and, as a result, that her recovery would be quick and complete.

In addition, Betsy conditioned her subconscious mind with daily affirmations, developing the optimistic belief that the surgery would go well and that her recovery would be rapid. After her operation, she followed the recommendations of her physical therapist, mainly to *Keep Moving,* albeit slowly at first. She recited her affirmation, "I'm getting better every day in every way," throughout each day. I reinforced her optimism by pointing out ways in which she improved day by day, such as walking more upright.

Her operation was a resounding success. I have no data to ascertain how much of her success arose from her positive mindset, but I can't imagine that it impeded her recovery.

preventing accidents, and (7) getting regular checkups. All seven health behaviors were significantly positively correlated with optimism. Therefore, developing positive emotions such as optimism and setting goals relating to good health might help older Americans make better choices that lead to improved health and well-being[36].

Further evidence shows that positive self-perceptions of aging are associated with greater adoption of preventive health behaviors[17]. In 1975, participants in a study of aging and retirement were asked a series of questions regarding their belief about aging. In 1995, participants still in the study were asked whether they employed eight preventive health behaviors on a five-point scale ranging from "never" to "always." Participants with a positive self-perception of aging in 1975 employed significantly more positive health behaviors 20 years later than participants with a negative self-perception, after adjustment for confounding factors. Thus, improving our self-perceptions of aging might be an effective way to maintain or improve our health as we age[37].

Increased well-being

Religious traditions have long exhorted people to be grateful. The state of gratitude is valuable in its own right and may lead to other positive outcomes. Yet, until recently, the contribution of gratitude to health and well-being was speculative, lacking empirical verification. In an effort to increase the rigor of gratitude studies, Robert Emmons and Michael McCullough conducted three related controlled experiments that investigated the effects of gratitude on aspects of psychological and physical well-being. University students served as research subjects in two experiments, while adults with neuromuscular disease participated in a third. In these studies, subjects were randomly assigned to one of four groups (depending on the study): gratitude, hassle, downward social comparison, and control. The gratitude experiments ran for either 10, 13, or 21 weeks.

The results of the studies supported the popular view that focusing on our blessings improves well-being. In study 1, students in the gratitude intervention rated their life more favorably, had more optimism for the upcoming week, and had fewer symptoms of physical illness than students in the other two groups. In study 2, students in the gratitude group reported greater positive affect and a greater sense of connectedness to others than those in the hassle or downward social comparison groups. In study 3, the gratitude intervention led to higher scores for positive affect, sleep quality and amount, and a better scores for negative affect compared members of the control group. Overall, inducing a state of gratefulness through gratitude exercises created varying emotional, physical, and interpersonal benefits. These findings remind us that gratitude may build enduring psychological, social, and spiritual resources that we can draw upon in difficult times[38].

Gratitude may also promote psychological well-being in persons with chronic medical conditions. A recent longitudinal study addressed this issue with respect to depression in patients with either of two chronic conditions: arthritis and inflammatory bowel disease (IBD). Patients with arthritis (423) and IBD (427) completed online surveys at baseline. One hundred sixty-three people with arthritis and 144 people with IBD completed the follow-up survey six months later. Higher gratitude at baseline was associated with less depressive symptoms at both baseline and six months in both arthritis and IBD patients. Gratitude at baseline remained a significant and unique predictor of lower depression at six months after controlling for other relevant variables in both sets of patients. Therefore, even if we have a chronic disease, being grateful may promote psychological well-being[39].

Greater use of preventive health services

Positive self-perceptions lead older adults to increase their use of preventive health services. Results from a sample of 6,177 people in the 2008 wave of the Health and Retirement Study showed that aging satisfaction was significantly associated with greater use of mammograms, Pap smears, prostate exams, and other health services. Prior research showed that adults who believed that health problems were inevitable in older age were less likely to engage in preventive health behaviors[40]. Studies also show that people who attribute having a heart attack or stroke to their age, as opposed to lifestyle choices, are less likely to make better lifestyle choices after the event[40]. On a behavioral level, positive self-perceptions predict more preventive health behaviors in older adults[36] and maintenance of health status over time[42].

Reduced risk of cognitive impairment

Higher levels of dispositional optimism have been associated with behaviors and biological processes that support mental health. Researchers recently investigated the relationship between optimism and cognitive impairment using data from 4,624 participants aged 65 or older from the 2006 wave of the Health and Retirement Study. Compared to participants ranked in the lowest one-third of optimism, participants ranked in the highest one-third had a 4 to 52 percent lower risk of developing cognitive impairment, depending on which statistical model was used. Furthermore, the risk of developing cognitive impairment declined in a graded manner as the level of optimism increased, suggesting that higher optimism might cause a reduced risk of cognitive decline. Perhaps optimistic people can self-regulate better than pessimistic people and engage in better problem solving. Also, optimistic people are more likely to seek social support, which protects against cognitive decline. Happily, studies show that optimism can be learned. Greater optimism, if widely learned through the U.S., might substantially reduce the incidence of cognitive impairment over time[43].

Faster recovery from disability

Disability is a major issue for older people because it can seriously compromise their quality of life. Why do some people recover much faster than others from similar disabilities? Self-perception of aging may explain, at least partially, varying rates of recovery for different people. Researchers used data from a project that recruited people from the greater New Haven, Connecticut, area. The participants (aged 70 or older at baseline) were interviewed monthly for up to 129 months and completed home-based assessments of disability and various physical and mental factors every 18 months. Compared to the negative-age-stereotype group, the positive-age-stereotype group had a 44 percent greater likelihood to recover completely from severe disability. Furthermore, people in the positive-age-stereotype group showed a slower rate of decline in their ability to engage in activities of daily living[44]. Our beliefs and attitudes profoundly impact our life experience. Shifting from a negative- to a positive-age-stereo-type appears to increase our well-being.

Healthy aging

Optimism extends to heathy aging. Data from 33,326 women (average age of 68 at baseline) followed for eight years as part of the Nurses' Health Study provide evidence. "Healthy aging" was defined as exhibiting the following categories at the end of the follow-up: (1) remaining free of major chronic diseases, (2) having no subjective memory impairment, (3) having intact physical function, and (4) surviving through follow-up. Greater optimism predicted better measures of healthy aging. Compared to participants in the lowest quartile of optimism, those in the highest quartile had a 23 percent greater likelihood of achieving healthy aging. The odds of achieving healthy aging increased as optimism increased and more strongly in the upper three quartiles of optimism scores. Being more optimistic may improve our prospects of healthy aging[45].

Poor Outcomes Linked to Failing to *Develop a Positive Mental Attitude*

Chronic negative thoughts and emotions can affect us in more ways than we might realize. Research shows that people who fail to *Develop a Positive Mental Attitude* are not only less happy, but they are more likely to experience undesirable physical and mental health outcomes.

Bad Outcomes Linked to Failing to *Develop a Positive Mental Attitude*	Premature death Cardiac events Hypertension Markers of inflammation Increased risk of depression and anxiety Walking more slowly

Premature death

A representative sample of 6,928 people in Alameda County, California, who rated their health as poor in 1965 had a two-fold higher rate of mortality over the next nine years, compared to those who rated their health as excellent. Here's the kicker: perceived health was not related to one's objective physical health status. Thus, it appears that our thoughts, beliefs, and attitudes about our health can affect our longevity, regardless of our physical health[46].

It would seem that people who don't enjoy life (perhaps as a consequence of a negative or pessimistic mental attitude) wouldn't live as long as those who enjoy life. Japanese researchers tested this idea with data from 88,175 Japanese men and women aged 40–69 at baseline and followed over an average of 12 years. Men with low perceived enjoyment of life had a multivariable-adjusted greater risk of dying from coronary heart disease (91 percent higher), stroke (86 percent higher), all types of cardiovascular disease combined (62 percent higher), and had a greater risk of developing any type of cardiovascular disease (272 percent higher) compared to men with a high enjoyment of life. Perceived enjoyment of life in women was not significantly associated with risk of any cause of mortality or any type of cardiovascular disease. At least for Japanese men, a pessimistic mental attitude predicted a greater risk of premature death from cardiovascular disease and greater harm to their cardiovascular health[47].

Stereotypic views regarding older people often include negative statements such as, "Old age is a dreary time of life." In fact, studies show that negative beliefs about aging predict negative health outcomes among older adults. Researchers recently extended previous studies using data from 105 elderly, community-dwelling Canadians aged 80 or older. Subjects who scored high on attributing chronic diseases to "old age" had poorer health symptoms, poorer health maintenance behaviors, and a 60 percent higher risk of dying after two years of follow-up, compared to those who scored low. Older people who attribute chronic illness to old age may subconsciously act in ways that make this belief come true. Alternatively, we can adopt the belief that old age can be a time of vibrant health and well-being. Our subconscious mind will tend to direct us to act in ways to make this belief come true[48].

Cardiac events

Research shows that people who hold a negative-age-stereotype are more likely to experience a cardiac event (any incident that may damage the heart) than those with a positive-age stereotype. Stereotypes from our surrounding culture become embodied earlier in life when we accept the stereotypes as self-defining[49].

Data from the Baltimore Longitudinal Study on Aging support the idea that age stereotypes created earlier in life impact health and well-being later in life. Researchers collected information from participants who were age 49 or younger at baseline in 1968 and had no prior cardiovascular events. Younger individuals who held more negative-age stereotypes were 8 percent more likely to have a cardiac event during the ensuing 38 years compared to those who held more positive-age stereotypes. While the difference was small, it was statistically significant. Moreover, at every time point at which data were collected, those with a negative-age stereotype were more likely to experience a cardiac event than those with a positive-age stereotype[50].

Hypertension

Hypertension is defined as systolic blood pressure of 140 or higher and a diastolic blood pressure of 90 or higher. High blood pressure predicts a higher risk of cardiovascular disease than lower blood pressure, and its prevalence increases with age. A 1985 study sought to shed more light on hypertension early in adult life in relation to psychosocial factors including time urgency/impatience, achievement/striving, hostility, depression, and anxiety. The sample included 3,308 African-American and white adults ages 18–30, recruited from four U.S. metropolitan areas, and followed for approximately 15 years. Time urgency/impatience and achievement/striving were significantly associated with the risk of developing hypertension at 15 years post-baseline. Compared with those in the lowest quartile, the risk of developing hypertension for those in the highest quartile of scores for both time urgency/impatience and hostility was 184 percent higher. The increase in risk for those in the highest quartile of scores for urgency/impatience increased in a graded manner as scores increased, suggesting a cause-and-effect relationship, especially for white men. No significant relationship appeared between hypertension and achievement/striving, depression, or anxiety. Thus, young adults, especially white men, would likely benefit from reducing their tendency to react to life's circumstances with time urgency/impatience or hostility[51].

Markers of inflammation

Recent evidence suggests that both optimism and pessimism are associated with several positive and negative aspects, respectively, of cardiovascular disease. Yet the mechanisms that underlie these associations remain fuzzy. A recent study addressed this situation by investigating the associations between optimism and pessimism and seven markers of inflammation and blood clotting. Data were taken from 6,814 American men and women aged 45–84 years who participated in the Multi-Ethnic Study of Atherosclerosis. A more positive disposition predicted significantly lower concentrations of three of the four markers of inflammation (interleukin-6, fibrinogen, and homocysteine, but not C-reactive protein) and none of the three markers of blood clotting (D-dimer, factor VIII, and PAP). Scores on the optimism subscale were not significantly associated with any of the seven markers. However, scores on the pessimism subscale were significantly associated with all four markers of inflammation but none of the three markers of blood clotting. The strength of the associations of pessimism with inflammatory markers was similar to those observed for an increase in age of ten years[52].

Increased risk of depression and anxiety

Depression later in life predicts a greater risk of suicide, cognitive impairment, and impaired social functioning; the effects of anxiety are similar. Researchers used data from the Irish Longitudinal Study on Aging to investigate the association between negative perceptions of aging and the onset and persistence of depression. The nationally representative sample of Irish adults included 6,095 subjects with a minimum age of 50 at baseline. Negative perceptions of aging during Wave 1 (2009-2011) were associated with the onset of depression and anxiety during Wave 2 (2012-2013). A one-point increase in the baseline negative-aging-perception scale (which ranged from 1-5) predicted a 9 and 4 percent increased risk of depression and anxiety, respectively. Subjects with negative perceptions of aging and who exhibited depression or anxiety during Wave 1 were more likely to remain depressed or anxious during Wave 2.

Negative perceptions of aging could combine with perceptions of low control over the aging process and the prospect of poorer health in the future, causing older people to avoid preventive and health-promoting actions. In addition, people with negative perceptions of aging might not seek help for depression or anxiety, thinking that psychological distress is an inevitable part of aging. People may experience negative-aging stereotypes as environmental stressors, which may further compound their depression and anxiety. Changing our perceptions of aging from negative to positive could improve our mental health[53].

Walking more slowly

Walking speed is a reliable measure of physical function in older people. Irish and British researchers recently investigated whether negative perceptions of aging were related to long-term declines in walking speed. The researchers used data from 3,913 relatively healthy subjects (average age of 63 years) in the Irish Longitudinal Study on Aging. The average follow-up period was 24 months. Subjects who expressed stronger beliefs in a lack of control and the negative consequences of aging had a greater decline in walking speed than those who did not. Feelings of a lack of control and expectations of negative outcomes may lead to decreased feelings of self-efficacy and, over time, decreased health-maintenance behaviors. This and other studies found harmful effects of believing—consciously or unconsciously—that aging is negative. Failing to *Develop a Positive Mental Attitude* about aging may diminish our *Quality of Lifespan*[54].

Practical Ways to *Develop a Positive Mental Attitude*

Each of us is endowed with a predisposition for a certain mental attitude. But researchers have demonstrated through controlled experiments that we can learn to improve our mental attitude. We can purge our vocabulary of negative self-talk and self-limiting phrases. We can develop attitudes of optimism, gratitude, forgiveness, and positivity.

By nature, I believe I have a positive mental attitude. But I have developed even greater optimism, positivity, gratitude, and forgiveness by following the suggestions below. As a consequence, I feel I am a healthier and happier person.

- **Replace negative self-perceptions of aging with positive self-perceptions.** The following exercise, designed to increase positive stereotypes of aging, is based on one developed by Becca Levy and colleagues[55].

Reflect on Words that Support Positive Aging Stereotypes

1. Write one of the words below on a sticky note and post it in a place where you'll see it frequently—such as on your refrigerator or your bathroom mirror:

   Accomplished Astute Capable Careful Competent Considerate Courteous Enlightened Experienced Gracious Learned Intelligent Judicious Perceptive Proficient Prudent Qualified Sensible Skilled Tactful Thoughtful Wise

2. When you see the word, reflect for a moment on your feelings about it. Leave the word in place for a week, then replace the sticky note with one with a different word from the list above written on it. Over 23 weeks, you'll be primed daily with positive-age stereotypes.

- **Cultivate a sense of gratitude.** Musing on gratitude can help us savor life's experiences and help us derive maximum satisfaction from them. Focusing on our blessings may counter our tendency to take positive things in our lives, such as a new car, for granted[56]. Developing a sense of gratitude involves thinking and writing about the many things in life, both large and small, for which we can be grateful. These might include supportive relationships, sacrifices or contributions others have made for us, or facts about our life, such as our advantages and opportunities. In all these cases, we can identify previously unappreciated aspects of our life for which we can be thankful.

   The following two exercises can help you develop a sense of gratitude. The act of writing will help you focus on what you have and the possibilities in your life rather than on what you don't have and what isn't working.

Think of Things for Which You Are Grateful

1. Each Sunday evening over the next three months, think of five things from the preceding week for which you are grateful and write them down.
2. Think of what might have caused each of the five things[38.]

Keep a Gratitude Journal

1. Buy a small bound book in which you can record your thoughts and feelings.
2. Every day, write down something for which you are grateful.
3. Contemplate how your life is more rewarding as a consequence of being grateful.

- **Reflect on your best possible self.** The best possible self exercise creates an immediate increase in positive affect and an immediate decrease in negative affect. Researchers in the Netherlands[57] used the following best possible self exercise. This exercise, followed over a two-week period, produced a significant increase in dispositional optimism, positive future events, and positive affect, as well as a significant decrease in negative future events and negative affect.

Best Possible Self

1. Think about your best possible self. Imagine a future in which everything has turned out as well as it could have. Imagine that you've worked diligently and have realized all your life goals. Envision satisfying all your life dreams and developing your potential to the fullest.
2. Now think about the best possible ways in which your life could develop in your personal, relational, and professional

domains. Thinking along these lines will help you make decisions in the present.

3. Keep thinking about and imagining yourself in this way during the next week.

4. To help you build your best possible self, write down your desires, the skills you want to develop, and the goals you want to achieve in the future for your personal, relational, and professional domains. Complete this part of the exercise in 20 minutes. Begin as many sentences as you can with the phrase, "In the future, I will…" Then merge what you've written about the three domains into a coherent personal story—as you might write in a diary—that you'd like to read some day.

5. When you're done, spend five minutes visualizing your story in as much vivid detail and with as much emotion as possible.

6. Repeat the five-minute visualization exercise once a day over the next week.

- **Acknowledge the good things in your life.** The following two exercises will help you recognize good things in your life and about yourself[58].

Three Good Things in Life

1. Every evening over the next week, write down three things that went well each day.

2. Reflect on what caused each thing to turn out well and write that down.

Using Character Strengths in a New Way

1. Go online to Via Character
   (http://www.viacharacter.org/www/Character-Strengths-Survey) and complete the free character strengths survey to discover your best qualities.
2. Over the next week, use one of your top character strengths in a new and different way.
3. Spend a few minutes each evening reflecting on what you experienced.

- **Learn to forgive.** Spending your mental and emotional energy on the positive things in your life helps you shift that energy away from grievance stories. Fred Luskin offers a number of practical forgiveness suggestions in his book *Forgive for Good*[13]. I strongly recommend buying the book and doing the exercises. Luskin offers two techniques as presented in the following exercises to help you reclaim responsibility for your feelings.

Remind Yourself of the Good Things in Your Life

1. If you have visited great scenic wonders, such as the Grand Canyon or Yosemite Valley, consciously refocus your mind on the delightful experience. You are in charge of deciding where your attention will go.
2. Choose an uplifting topic, such as beauty, gratitude, or love, and relax into a positive experience that you've had in one of those realms or in another one that's equally appealing.

Positive Emotion Refocusing Technique

1. Relax with several deep breaths.
2. Visualize a beautiful scene perhaps in nature or in an elegantly designed building or an inviting room.
3. Imagine warm feelings surrounding your heart.
4. Ask your relaxed and peaceful self what you can do to resolve your difficulty.

- **Practice expressive writing.** People who don't express their feelings about an upsetting experience fail to translate their thoughts and feelings into language. It's essential to put a powerful emotional event into some kind of coherent story that has personal meaning, thereby reducing the need to think about it as much. Expressive writing seems to help people come to terms with a troubling event and put the event into a perspective that no longer elicits anxiety or shame. Expressive writing, developed by Jamie Pennebaker and Sandy Beall in 1986, has been applied to many different situations. Soldiers with post-traumatic stress disorder, women who have been raped, and persons who have lost their spouses to divorce or death have found relief through expressive writing[59]. Expressive writing involves relatively short amounts of time, such as 15 minutes per day for four consecutive days.

1. Take about 15 minutes each day for the next four days to write about your deepest emotions and thoughts concerning the most upsetting experience in your life. Let go and explore your feelings and thoughts about it. In your writing, you might tie this experience to your childhood, your relation-

ship with your parents, people whom you have loved, people you love now, or to your career. Reflect on how this experience relates to who you would like to become and who you have been in the past. If you not had a traumatic experience, you've undoubtedly experienced major conflicts or stressors. You can write about one of them as well. You can write about the same issue every day or a series of different issues. Whatever you choose to write about, it's critical that you really let go and explore your deepest emotions and thoughts.

2. After you finish writing, you may feel somewhat depressed or sad. That's understandable. As with seeing a sad movie, this typically goes away in a couple of hours. If you find you are getting extremely upset about a writing topic, simply stop writing or change topics until you are ready to approach the sensitive topic another time.

- **Walk in nature.** A recent study showed that mountain walking promoted positive mood and elation, while diminishing fatigue, depression, anger, and anxiety. This research mirrors other studies that show positive emotional responses to walking or otherwise being in nature[60]. Even if you don't have daily access to mountain scenery, spend more time outdoors in natural settings.

- **Mindfully control your emotions.** Matt Tennney offers the four-step SCIL (Stop, Control, Investigate, Look) method to practice mindfulness of emotions[61]. The following exercise will help you deal resourcefully with highly emotional situations.

Stop, Control, Investigate, Look

1. **Stop.** Taking a momentary timeout helps prevent emotions from consuming us. If you're particularly agitated, remove yourself for a few minutes from the emotional situation to allow you to calm down.

2. **Control the breath and name the emotion.** Intentionally slow your breathing and breathe more deeply. Controlling your breathing helps stop the fight-or-flight response. Naming the emotion and slowing the breath to return you to a positive emotional state quickly. For example, imagine that you're frustrated with your spouse who wants both of you to see a film that you heard got bad reviews. After moving through step 1 and controlling your breath, say silently to yourself in the in-breath, "There is frustration." On the out-breath say silently, "I handle frustration."

3. **Investigate the emotion like a mad scientist.** Once you calm down a bit, on the in-breath say silently to yourself, "There is frustration." On the out-breath say, "What is frustration like in the body?" Notice without judgment what frustration feels like in your body, while continuing the breathing patterns just described. What sensation(s) do you find yourself experiencing? Sometimes step 3 will be all that's necessary to reestablish mindfulness of emotions.

4. **Look deeply.** What caused the emotion(s) to erupt? Attempt to see the situation from the other person's perspective. For example, perhaps one of your spouse's friends recommended the film highly.

- **Associate with positive, upbeat, can-do people.** The people with whom we associate affect how we behave, the choices we make, and the life we experience. Even the associates of our associates appear to affect our lives positively or negatively[62].

Three Key Points

1. *Develop a Positive Mental Attitude*, and you will notably improve your emotional well-being.

2. Optimism, gratitude, and forgiveness are crucial aspects of a positive mental attitude.

3. You can learn to become more optimistic, grateful, and forgiving.

Chapter 8

Live with Purpose

Those who spend their time searching for happiness never find it, while those who search for meaning, purpose, and strong personal relationships find that happiness usually comes to them as a by-product of those three things.
—Nido Qubein

In his book *The Power of Purpose*, career coach and best-selling author Richard Leider defines living with purpose as "the aim around which we structure our lives, a source of direction and energy, and the way the meaning of our lives is worked out in daily experience"[1]. Martin Seligman, often called the father of positive psychology, states that a purposeful life creates meaning and achievement, two of the hallmarks of flourishing and well-being[2]. People who have life purpose tend to operate on a higher plane of existence than others.

Purpose can arise from several sources. We are fortunate if our daily work provides us with a sense of purpose. More importantly, purpose also arises from serving others. For Leider, service to others includes people, animals, plants, and the inanimate world. Service to others may involve volunteer work, helping elderly neighbors, and participating in community projects, among other things.

Research suggests that people who *Live With Purpose* are healthier, happier, and live longer. For example, those who *Live With Purpose* have a lower risk of cardiovascular disease, a lower risk of Alzheimer's disease, fewer sleep disturbances, and they make better use of preventive health services than people who don't *Live With Purpose.*

The value of living with purpose extends beyond better health. Teresa Amabile of the Harvard Business School and psychologist Steven Kramer found that the most powerful influence on whether employees in the corporate world experience a satisfying inner life is progress in meaningful work[3]. A recent book, *The Future-Proof Workplace* by Linda Sharkey and Morag Barrett[4], makes the case that, in the business world, purpose (stated in compelling phrases and actually embraced) is replacing mission and vision (stated in polished phrases and usually ignored) as a bedrock of a successful enterprise.

About 35 years ago, Claire Nuer developed a set of personal mastery tools to "help build sustainable personal and organizational change". The organizational consulting firm, Learning as Leadership, grew out of Claire Nuer's work; her daughter, Lara, continues Claire's work today. Two aspects of the Learning as Leadership approach apply to creating lifelong health and well-being. One aspect is called "Taking Stock of the Past," which includes asking ourselves difficult questions about our past choices in order to make informed decisions about our health and well-being going forward. For instance: Has my previous behavior led me to a place I want to be? If not, where would I rather be? The other aspect is "Taking Action in the Present." The Nuers propose setting a noble goal as part of one's personal mastery. A noble goal is one that has an overarching purpose that extends beyond individual goals of material gain or success. The primary recipients include "loved ones, colleagues, the community, and the planet." Thus, living with purpose not only supports our own health and well-being, but also that of the wider world[5].

Karl Pillemer, in his book *30 Lessons for Living*, poses this question: Do I wake up in the morning looking forward to work? In a broader sense, he could have asked: Do I wake up in the morning looking forward to living? Making purposeful choices every day helps us find meaning and fulfillment in life[6].

Benefits Linked to *Live with Purpose*

"Higher levels of meaning are clearly associated with better physical health, as well as behavioral factors that decrease the probability of negative health outcomes or increase that of positive health outcomes." This was the conclusion by the authors of a 2014 review of 70 published scientific studies. Improved negative health behaviors included less binge eating, reduced risk of smoking, and lower risk of relapse following drug or smoking cessation. Greater health-promoting behaviors included more exercise, better eating, better sleep, greater relaxation, regular breast cancer self-exams, and greater self-efficacy[7].

This section highlights the multiple potential benefits of *Live with Purpose* and the scientific research that supports them. As a consequence of living with purpose, we can bring more meaning to our lives and extend our *Quality of Lifespan*.

Benefits linked to *Live with Purpose*
- Increased longevity
- Better cardiovascular health
- Better overall health
- Better mental health
- Better cognitive function later in life
- Greater well-being
- Greater use of preventive health services, less hospitalization
- Greater physical function later in life
- Increased self-efficacy
- Better eating habits and increased physical activity
- Fewer sleep disturbances
- Greater likelihood of post-traumatic growth

Increased longevity

A 2014 study found that purposeful U.S. adults who were followed over a 14-year period lived longer than nonpurposeful adults, even after accounting for characteristics of psychological and affective well-being. In addition, longer life span did not depend on the subjects' age or whether they had retired or not. The researchers concluded that, "having a purpose in life appears to widely buffer against mortality risk across the adult years[8].

Purposeful activities can be mundane and still predict increased longevity. In a classic study, psychologists Ellen Langer and Judith Rodin wanted to know how a sense of control might affect the lives of 91 nursing home patients. Just over half of the patients were given a potted plant and asked to care for it. The other participants were also given a potted plant but were told that the nursing home staff would care for it. Eighteen months after the initial study, the researchers returned to the nursing home to determine how the patients fared. Rodin and Langer found that the nursing home staff judged that patients who took care of their plants were significantly more actively engaged, more sociable, and more vigorous than patients who did not care for their plants. Surprisingly, given the age and physical condition of the nursing home residents, the health ratings of the patients who took care of their plants improved over the next 18 months, while those of the other patients declined. Finally, only 15 percent of the patients who took care of their plants died over the 18 months compared to 30 percent of the other patients. These outcomes suggest that declining health, even in institutionalized elderly patients, can be slowed or possibly reversed over 18 months. In addition, it appears that some combination of increased sense of control over one's life and increased purposeful activity promotes better health and longevity in elderly persons[9]. If simply caring for a potted plant could increase our longevity, imagine what a fully purposeful life could do in terms of making our lives more worth living and extending our *Quality of Lifespan.*

Volunteering Predicts Lower Mortality Risk

Volunteering can be a purposeful activity. A new meta-analysis of 14 studies focused on organized volunteer activities by older adults (age 55 and up). The results showed that volunteering predicted 47 percent and 24 percent reductions in death rate when confounding factors were excluded and included, respectively. A reduced risk of premature death may arise, at least in part, by providing volunteers with a sense of purpose and opportunities to develop social support. Organized volunteering appears to be a win-win situation for both volunteer and recipient. The authors stated that "it is no longer a question of whether volunteering is predictive of mortality risk; our results suggest that the association is reliable, and that the magnitude of the relationship is sizeable[10]."

Another study found that elderly people who engage in social and productive activities may live longer than those who don't engage in such activities. Data collection for the New Haven, Connecticut, Epidemiological Studies of the Elderly began in 1982. The cohort at baseline included 2,812 women and men age 65 and older living in the community. Over the next 13 years, 62 percent of the cohort died. Social, productive, and fitness activities all significantly and independently predicted lower mortality in a graded manner. Mortality was the lowest for individuals in the highest category of productive activity, while mortality was highest for people in the lowest category of productive activity. Social and productive activities may create a sense of meaning and purpose in life, which in turn may promote greater longevity[11].

If meaning in life predicts a longer lifespan, does the benefit arise indirectly, perhaps by increasing healthy choices or immune function? Neal Krause at the University of Michigan used data from a nationwide survey of adults 65 and older to address this question. More specifically, he analyzed data from participants in Waves 4 (2002–2003), 5 (2005), and 6 (2007). In Wave 4, meaning in life was significantly positively associated with education, being married, self-rated health, and emotional support, and negatively associated with age, serious illness, non-serious illness, and functional disability. Using data from all the waves, meaning in life was significantly negatively associated with mortality. But when potential confounding effects (self-reported health, serious illness, non-serious illness, and functional disability) were added to the statistical model, the effect of meaning on mortality became statistically nonsignificant. Evidently, the effect of meaning in life on mortality operated indirectly by promoting aspects of better physical health. Of the four dimensions of meaning in life investigated in this study—purpose, values, goals, and reconciling the past—purpose had the strongest association with increased longevity[12].

Purpose in life contributes to well-being, which can be parsed into three subsets: (1) life satisfaction; (2) feelings of happiness, anger, stress, pain; and (3) a sense of purpose/meaning in life, also known as eudemonic well-being. Researchers analyzed data for 9,050 participants (average age 65 years) who were followed for an average of eight years in the English Longitudinal Study of Ageing. Survival during the follow-up period increased progressively by nine, 13, 18, and 29 percent, respectively, for participants in the lowest through the highest quartiles of eudemonic well-being. After controlling for confounding factors, participants in the highest quartile of eudemonic well-being had a 30 percent lower risk of dying over 8 years compared to participants in the lowest quartile. While epidemiological data such as these do not prove cause-and-effect, the graded nature of observed mortality with decreasing eudemonic well-being points toward a causal relationship[13]. On average, people who lived with purpose lived longer than those who didn't.

A Sense of Control May Lead to Longer Lifespan

Studies have examined the link between purpose in life and health, but none have explored which living with purpose pathways might lead people to make healthy choices over time. A recent study, using data from a large national survey of Americans over a 10-year period, did just that. The researchers used the outcome measure of allostatic load, defined as the physiological effects from repeated or chronic challenges the body experiences as stressful. Allostatic load is measured by various indicators that reflect cumulative strain on the body. The study revealed that purpose in life was significantly negatively correlated with several indicators of allostatic load: lipid metabolism, glucose metabolism, and parasympathetic nervous system activity. Purpose in life at Wave 1 (1995–1996) and age at baseline predicted total allostatic load. Those participants who had a higher perceived sense of control over their own health had a lower allostatic load. Thus, having a sense of greater control over one's own health mediated part of the inverse relationship between purpose in life and allostatic load. Therefore, both living with purpose and having a greater sense of control over our health may increase longevity[14].

Better cardiovascular health

According to the Centers for Disease Control[15], stroke was the fifth leading cause of death in the U.S. in 2015. Recent research shows that purpose in life predicts the occurrence of cardiovascular diseases, potentially including stroke. Researchers used data from the Health and Retirement Study, a nationally representative study, for 6,739 American adults over the age of 50 who were stroke-free at baseline. Over a four-year follow-up period, greater baseline purpose in life predicted a significantly reduced risk of stroke for these older Americans, after adjusting for age, gender, race/ethnicity, marital status, education level, total wealth, functional status, biological factors, and psychological factors[16].

In other research efforts, scientists systematically searched databases of studies regarding the relationship between purpose in life, mortality, and cardiovascular events. Ten prospective studies with a total of 136,265 participants formed the analysis. A higher purpose in life predicted a 17 percent reduction in all-cause mortality and cardiovascular events. Results were similar across different questionnaires used to measure purpose in life, various countries of origin, different ages, and

Student Volunteers Have Decreased Cardiovascular Risk

Researchers recently designed a randomized, controlled trial to see if volunteering activity by adolescents would improve their cardiovascular risk factors.

Subjects included 90 sophomores at an urban high school in western Canada. The students were randomly assigned to either a volunteer group or a control group, members of which were wait-listed to volunteer later in the school year. Students in the volunteer group helped students at a nearby elementary school with various activities (such as homework, sports programs, and cooking) after school for 1–1.5 hours per week for 10 weeks.

At the end of the 10-week period, the volunteering group showed significantly lower body mass index, total cholesterol, and interleukin 6 (a marker of inflammation), while levels of C-reactive protein (another marker of inflammation) marginally declined. The control group exhibited no differences in these markers at the end of the 10-week period. Students in the volunteering group who increased most in empathy and altruistic behaviors and who decreased most in negative whether or not participants with baseline cardiovascular disease were included in the study. Thus, a high sense of purpose in life foretold a reduced risk for all-cause mortality and cardiovascular events[17].

Better overall health

Mounting evidence suggests that greater meaning in life is associated with better health-related outcomes, including making healthier choices, less cognitive decline, and reduced premature mortality. The reasons why meaning in life might be linked to positive health outcomes are less clear. Researchers used a sample of 571 college undergraduate students in a psychology class to test the proposition that having meaning in life leads to a more positive health orientation, which predicts more positive health outcomes. The researchers found that having meaning in life was related to better health. Furthermore, positive health orientation explained some of the effects of meaning in life on health symptoms. The findings more or less supported the authors' model of how meaning in life and proactive health orientation interact to support better health outcomes[19]. Intuitively, it makes sense that psychological variables such as greater meaning in life would promote health-related behaviors. Why would we make healthy choices if we didn't connect the consequences of making those choices to things that matter most to us in life?

While the health effects of volunteering are well-documented, it's not clear if those effects are associated with volunteer efforts that largely benefit oneself or others. Self-oriented volunteering might

mood had the greatest decreases in cardiovascular risk factors during the study[18].

Wouldn't it be great if we could do well by others while doing well by ourselves? That's exactly what this study shows. Imagine the potential upside if volunteering were to become part and parcel of the educational experience of young people. The benefits of volunteering likely accrue not only to the students being helped but also to the students doing the helping.

include service in political campaigns, environmental causes, or animal-related welfare. Other-oriented volunteering might include service in education, health, or religious groups. A new study using data from the Survey of Texas Adults in 2004 showed that both types of volunteering had significant positive health effects, except for self-oriented volunteering on depression (no effect). Other-oriented volunteering predicted significantly stronger effects on mental and physical health outcomes, especially for social well-being. Volunteering appears to predict healthy living[20].

Better mental health

Limited research suggests that social interest—defined as a cooperative approach toward life and striving for an ideal community—and/or altruism are associated with better life adjustment, better marital adjustment, greater perceived meaning in life, less hopelessness, and better physical health. Helping others may partially explain the association between religious involvement and better self-reported health.

Emerging research indicates that altruistic or social interest behaviors may be advantageous for both the helper and the person receiving help. A study of members and clergy of the Presbyterian Church across the U.S. sought to determine if helping others was more beneficial than receiving help. A sample of 2,016 lay church leaders and pastors drawn from 425 congregations was used for the analysis. Both receiving help and giving help significantly predicted positive mental health.

Giving help is likely considered to be a purposeful activity by the persons providing it, thus helping them feel a sense of meaning in life. Giving help had a stronger effect than receiving help. Even though the givers in the study had a high overall level of mental health and physical function, the givers still benefitted more that the recipients. However, giving help to the point of being overwhelmed had a significant negative effect on the mental health of the giver[21].

Better cognitive function later in life

Researchers in Chicago investigated the connection between life purpose and Alzheimer's disease using data from 951 older persons (average age 80 years) who participated in the Memory and Aging Project at the Rush Medical Center. Volunteers recruited from local retirement centers and subsidized senior housing projects underwent initial evaluations for Alzheimer's disease, mild cognitive impairment, cognition, and purpose in life at baseline. The evaluations were repeated annually for up to seven years. The researchers found that participants without dementia at baseline but who developed Alzheimer's disease or mild cognitive impairment during follow-up reported lower life purpose than those who did not develop the disease or impairment during follow-up, regardless of other factors. Persons with greater life purpose at baseline had higher cognition and it declined less rapidly for those who had lower life purpose at baseline. Because purpose in life is potentially modifiable, older people could increase their sense of life purpose and potentially lower their risk of developing cognitive problems[22].

Other studies at the Rush Medical Center addressed whether purpose in life can modify the effect of Alzheimer's disease pathologies—amyloid plaques and neurofibrillary tangles—on cognitive function. Two hundred forty-six elderly persons (average age 88 years) who participated in the Memory and Aging Project consented to donate their brains for autopsy following their death. Purpose in life modified the association between a global measure of Alzheimer's disease pathology and cognition. People with higher levels of life purpose had better cognitive function and slower rates of cognitive decline with age than people with lower levels of life purpose. Greater life purpose also reduced the association between neurofibrillary tangles and cognition. The bottom line: Higher levels of life purpose may reduce the impact of Alzheimer's disease pathology on cognition in elderly persons[23].

Greater well-being

Nancy Morrow-Howell at Washington University in St. Louis and colleagues used nationally representative data from 3,617 subjects over age 60 in the Americans' Changing Lives study to better understand the positive relationship between volunteering and well-being. Well-being included three aspects: (1) self-rated health, (2) functional dependency, and (3) depression. In this sample, 34 percent of the subjects volunteered an average of 72 hours per year. Older adult volunteers who reported lots of volunteer hours—up to about 100 hours per year—reported higher levels of well-being than non-volunteers. Neither the number of organizations for which subjects volunteered, the type of organization, nor the perceived benefit to others predicted the well-being of volunteers. The simple act of volunteering itself appeared to be the most important predictor of subsequent well-being[24].

Americans aren't the only people to experience better health and well-being from volunteering. In Singapore, data were collected on 2,761 subjects 55 years or older at baseline, and on 1,754 of them two years later. Eighty-eight percent of the subjects were retired—of which 10 percent were volunteering, and 78 percent were not volunteering—with 12 percent still working. At baseline, the retired non-volunteering subjects scored worse on depression, cognitive status, positive mental well-being, and life satisfaction than their retired volunteering counterparts. At follow-up, non-volunteering subjects had worse scores on depression, cognitive status, and positive mental well-being than still-working subjects. This study supported a consistent and robust relationship between positive mental well-being and active work engagement or volunteer activities of retirees. The cognitive effect appeared to be greater in older (more than 62 years) than younger retirees[25]. *Live with Purpose* operating through work and volunteer activities may promote the cognitive health of older persons by providing opportunities for mental stimulation and new learning, thereby promoting successful aging.

An authentic happiness website developed by Martin Seligman invited responses from users regarding meaning in life, search for meaning in life, and how both relate to measures of well-being over one's life span. Responses were analyzed from 8,756 users of the website from November 2003 to February 2005. Users were grouped into four age classes: 18–24, 25–44, 45–64, and 65 and older. Meaning in life was correlated with well-being, with medium to large effect sizes that were highest for the two oldest age groups. Meaning in life was positively associated with happiness, positive affect, pleasure orientation, engagement orientation, and meaning orientation, and negatively associated with negative affect and depression. Within each age group, meaning orientation always had the greatest effect size. The search for meaning predicted lower life satisfaction, happiness, and positive affect and higher depression. This study suggests that older people are more able than younger people to make sense of their lives, even given declining physical capability and changing life roles. Older people may actively seek more opportunities to engage in life than previously thought[26].

Greater use of preventive health services, less hospitalization

The burgeoning population of American seniors predicts increased medical care expenses for those citizens along with major adverse economic consequences for the U.S. A recent analysis showed that annual medical care expenditures were 2.5 times higher per capita for Americans age 65 and older compared to people below age 65[27]. Americans over age 65 accounted for 41 percent of hospital expenses but made up only 14 percent of the U.S. population. Yet less than half of Americans over age 65 are up to date on basic preventive services.

To learn whether seniors who have greater purpose in life tend to make greater use of preventive health services, researchers used data over a six-year period from the Health and Retirement Study. After adjusting for sociodemographic factors, each one-unit increase in purpose (on a six-point scale) predicted a significantly greater likelihood that a participant would get a cholesterol test (18 percent increase), mammogram (27 percent increase), Pap smear (16 percent increase), or prostate examination (35 percent increase). Similarly, each one-unit increase in purpose predicted a 17 percent reduction in nights spent in a hospital. Participants in the top one-third of purpose spent 33 percent fewer nights in a hospital compared to those in the bottom one-third of purpose. If seniors increase their purpose in life, they may make better use of preventive measures, reduce their medical care expenses, and help the U.S. medical care system avoid bankruptcy[28].

Another study used data from the Health and Retirement Study to investigate whether volunteering is associated with the greater rates of preventive health care services or lower rates of hospitalization. In 2006, the Health and Retirement Study collected data on volunteer participation, as well as health-related information, including use of preventive services and rates of doctor and hospital visits. People who volunteered used preventive health services at higher rates, ranging from 21 to 53 percent, than people who didn't volunteer. People who volunteered had 38 percent fewer hospital visits compared to people who didn't volunteer. Those of us who volunteer may make more use of preventive services and have a lower rate of hospitalization[29].

Greater physical function later in life

Purpose in life predicts certain positive health behaviors and biological processes that may protect against declining physical function. Thus, greater purpose in life may indirectly reduce the risk of weak grip strength and slow walking speed. Researchers at Harvard investigated whether higher purpose in life among older adults predicted a lower risk of developing weak grip strength and slow walking speed over time. Both weak grip strength and slow walking speed are linked to declining physical function. Longitudinal data from the Health and Retirement Study were collected in 2006 and again in 2010. Researchers evaluated grip strength using spring-type hand dynamometers and walking speed with subjects walking 2.5 meters at their normal pace. After four years, and after controlling for multiple confounding factors, each standard deviation increase in purpose was significantly associated with an 11 percent lower risk of developing weak grip strength and a 9 percent decreased risk of developing slow walking speed. A sense of purpose in life may help older adults maintain physical function[30].

Increased self-efficacy

Self-efficacy refers to the feeling or belief that one has the ability to perform a specific action or succeed in a situation. Increased self-efficacy predicts a greater willingness to adopt healthy choices.

A common reason people cite for not engaging in healthy behaviors is lack of time. The following probably sounds familiar: "I'm too busy to volunteer at the local food pantry, even though I know it would help other people." Three business school researchers recently conducted experiments that reached a surprising conclusion: giving our time to others can increase the amount of time that we perceive we have. In one experiment, college students were randomly assigned to one of two groups. Students in one group spent five minutes writing an encouraging note to a gravely ill child, while students in the other group spent five minutes counting the letter "e" in pages of Latin text. Students who gave of their time by writing letters reported that they had more time than those who counted the letter "e."

In another experiment, participants recruited online were randomly assigned to one of two groups. Those in one group were asked to spend 30 minutes doing something previously unplanned for someone else. Those in the other group were asked to spend 10 minutes doing something unplanned for themselves. Participants who spent 30 minutes doing something for someone else perceived that they had more time than participants who spent 10 minutes on themselves. In a third experiment, college students in a laboratory session were told that the final 15 minutes of class would be spent on editing research essays written by at-risk students at a local high school. Half of the students were given essays and red pens for editing, while the rest were told that all the essays had already been edited and they could leave class early. As in the previous experiments, students who edited the essays reported having more spare time and that their time was less scarce, compared to the students who left class early and objectively had more time available.

A final experiment investigated possible mechanisms for the finding that giving away time increased the amount of perceived time available. Participants were recruited through Amazon's Mechanical Turk (a crowdsourcing marketplace). They were asked to vividly describe a recent expenditure of time doing something—either for themselves or someone else—that wasn't part of their ordinary routine. In addition, participants responded to statements that researchers used to evaluate self-efficacy, social connectedness, and meaningfulness. Participants who vividly described spending time on others reported having more time, greater self-efficacy, greater social connection, and greater meaning (but less enjoyment) than participants who described spending time on themselves. Analysis revealed that only self-efficacy mediated the effect of giving time on perceived time availability. Thus, giving time to others may increase our perceived amount of time available by increasing our own sense of self-efficacy[31].

Better eating and increased physical activity

A recent study of Romanian adolescents sheds new light on meaning in life and its associations with health behaviors. In this study, 456 Hungarian-speaking students (average age 18 years) in Romanian secondary schools formed the cohort. At baseline, the students filled out questionnaires relating to health-protective behaviors, valuing health, well-being, the presence of meaning in life, and the search for meaning in life. "The presence of meaning in life" referred to the degree to which students felt their lives were meaningful, and the "search for meaning in life" referred to the students' motivation to find or deepen the meaning in their lives. Health values, well-being, the presence of meaning, and the search for meaning all significantly predicted healthy eating and physical activity after 13 months for both boys and girls[32].

Fewer sleep disturbances

Sleep disturbances predict a range of adverse health problems, mental illness, and cognitive function. Older people are especially prone to sleep disturbances, with 40 to 70 percent reporting insomnia, disturbed sleep, or inadequate sleep. Researchers recently used data from the Health and Retirement Study to test the hypothesis that purpose in life predicts a reduced risk of sleep disturbances. Psychological and demographic data from 4,144 subjects who reported minimal or no sleep disturbances were collected at baseline in 2006. Follow-up sleep disturbances data were collected four years later. The researchers found that the likelihood of sleep disturbances declined as purpose in life increased. Each unit increase in life purpose on a six-point scale predicted a 16 percent reduced risk of sleep disturbances. This result might arise from more purposeful people adopting generally healthful behaviors that reduce the risk of sleep problems[34].

Greater likelihood of post-traumatic growth

Recent research confirms that trauma survivors can experience post-traumatic growth. A study of survivors of severe traumatic brain injury (TBI) investigated whether post-traumatic growth persists over a long period of time and what factors might predict post-traumatic growth. Twenty-one TBI survivors were interviewed and completed questionnaires that measured post-traumatic growth 11 and 13 years after injury. The researchers observed that the degree of post-traumatic

Increased Physical Activity Associated with Environmental Volunteering

Numerous studies have linked volunteering with positive physical and mental health outcomes in midlife and later. Surprisingly, research has minimally addressed the health outcomes of environmental volunteering, and until 2010 no longitudinal studies of the health effects of environmental volunteering had been reported. Researchers used data collected from a representative sample of 6,928 adults during 1965–1994 for the Alameda County Health Study. Statistical models showed that environmental volunteering was significantly associated with increased physical activity. Environmental volunteering in 1974 was also associated with a 45 percent lower risk of self-reported fair or poor physical health and a 51 percent lower risk of depression in 1994. Environmental volunteering predicted greater benefits than other types of volunteering[33].

Potential benefits of environmental volunteering include increased physical activity, increased sense of purpose, enhanced social integration, and enhanced psychological well-being due to greater connection with nature.

growth measured 11 years after injury did not change appreciably over the following two years. Thus, post-traumatic growth appeared to be relatively stable. Having a sense of personal meaning (purpose and coherence), high life satisfaction, social support, high activity levels, a high number of life events, paid work, new stable relationships after injury, milder disability, and religious faith were all significantly related to post-traumatic growth. Of these, a high level of life purpose was the best predictor of post-traumatic growth[35].

Given the trend of increasingly pervasive environmental problems and shrinking federal government budgets to address them on public lands in the U.S., environmental volunteering could be a win-win-win for the federal agencies, the environment, and the volunteers.

People who experience post-traumatic growth typically exhibit improvement in some or all of the following domains: personal strength, relating to others, appreciating life, new possibilities, and spiritual change. Post-traumatic growth can be regarded as a modern version of the long-established idea of redemption through suffering and denial. Abraham Maslow's concept of self-actualization and Carl Rogers' belief in the human tendency for self-actualization capture many of the beneficial features of post-traumatic growth. Thus, those who exhibit post-traumatic growth may achieve a higher level of flourishing. Post-traumatic growth likely involves active engagement with a traumatic experience and its consequences rather than denial or avoidance. Interestingly, the severity of the traumatic event is less important than a person's response to social, personal, and contextual variables[36]. A 2004 review of studies of disaster survivors found between 44 and 97 percent of survivors reported some positive aspects of post-traumatic growth. Experiences of psychological well-being associated with post-traumatic growth include autonomy, a sense of mastery, personal growth, positive relations with others, self-acceptance, and purpose in life[37].

Poor Outcomes Linked to Failing to *Live with Purpose*

Those of us who don't *Live with Purpose* are less likely to derive meaning and fulfillment from our lives. We also have higher risks of poor health outcomes.

Poor outcomes Linked to Failing to *Live with Purpose*	Premature death Decline in daily activities

Premature death

In Japan, *ikigai* is the most commonly used indicator of subjective well-being. *Ikigai* translates as "a sense of life worth living" or "a sense of well-being from being alive" or "purpose in life." Psychological factors, such as purpose in life, affect the risk of premature death. Thus, Japanese researchers used data from the Ohsaki National Health Insurance Cohort Study to determine if people who had *ikigai* had a lower risk of premature death. Over 40,000 research subjects from the Miyagi Prefecture in northeastern Japan were asked, "Do you have *ikigai* in your life?" Possible responses were yes, uncertain, or no. Compared to those who reported having *ikigai*, those who reported not having *ikigai* were more likely to be unmarried, unemployed, less educated, in poorer health, have a higher level of mental stress, have severe or moderate bodily pain, have limitations of physical function, and be less likely to walk at baseline. After seven years of follow-up, the risk of dying was 50 percent higher for those without *ikigai* compared to those with *ikigai*. In absolute terms, 93 percent of those having ikigai were still alive after seven years compared to 84 percent of those not having *ikigai*. After adjusting for age and sex, the risk of death due to cardiovascular disease, ischemic heart disease, stroke, pneumonia, and external causes were all significantly higher for those without *ikigai* compared to those with *ikigai*. For these Japanese residents, having a sense of purpose in life seemed to promote longer life[38].

We've all heard the expression "bored to death." Two British researchers (with perhaps too much time on their hands) wondered if that adage could literally be true. They used data from a study that followed 7,524 civil servants aged 35–55 living in London for 21–24 years. Participants were asked at baseline (from 1985-1988) if they were bored during the previous four weeks. Possible responses included a little, quite a bit, and a great deal. Participants who answered the question with "a great deal" had a 253 percent higher risk of cardiovascular mortality than those who responded with "not at all" during the follow-up period that ended in April 2009. Presumably, boredom as such was not the culprit. Rather, boredom likely served as a proxy for a lack of purpose and meaning in life and/or a shortage of supportive social relationships and attendant unhealthy behaviors such as drinking, smoking, and taking drugs. Thus, the healthy choices *Live with Purpose* and *Cultivate Social Connections* might counteract boredom and reduce the risk of premature death[39].

Decline in daily activities

Given the attention that some people devote to their hobbies, perhaps these activities might predict purpose and meaning in life. Hobbies might create meaning directly, especially for elderly people who no longer work. A trio of Japanese researchers hypothesized that community-dwelling elderly people who have a hobby and/or purpose in life (*ikigai*) would have a lower risk of premature death and a greater ability to perform activities of daily living, both regular (such as feeding, bathing, and grooming) and instrumental (such as using public transportation, preparing meals, and paying bills). The researchers studied 1,853 elderly people (mean age 76 years) in a rural Japanese town of about 6,900 residents from early 2011 to late 2014. Sixty-two percent of the participants stated that they had both hobbies and purpose in life. In all four statistical models used to analyze the data, having both hobbies and purpose in life predicted a lower risk of premature death. In the fully adjusted model, those with neither hobbies nor purpose in life had a *106 percent higher risk of dying* compared to those with both over nearly four years of follow-up. Participants with both hobbies and purpose showed a significantly lower risk of decline in instrumental activities of daily life compared to participants who had neither hobbies nor purpose. Those with purpose in life but not hobbies had an increased risk of decline in activities of daily living and instrumental activities of daily living compared to those with both. Thus, the combined lack of hobbies and purpose in life predicted greater risk of premature death and greater decline in activities of daily living for rural Japanese[40].

Practical Ways to *Live with Purpose*

- **Volunteer.** Thousands of volunteer opportunities exist in communities across the county and beyond. Your community may have a volunteer clearinghouse that can help you find a volunteer activity that suits you well.

- **Write a personal mission statement and a set of supporting goals.** Meaning in life has several characteristics, including a sense of coherence and order, the pursuit of worthwhile goals, and a sense that life is significant. While having meaning in life is associated with greater happiness, better health, and spiritual well-being, limited knowledge exists regarding *how* we can actually *Live with Purpose* and increase meaning in our life. Take some time to reflect and write about your long-term, overarching mission and goals that would support it. Brainstorm ways you can pursue them. This activity can help to strengthen and clarify your understanding of who you are, how you see the world, and how you fit into it[41].

- **Write expressively.** Living with purpose helps create meaning in life. Traumatic events that you don't satisfactorily resolve impede your ability to create meaning. People with unresolved traumatic events often ruminate about them, and in so doing perpetuate anxiety and other negative emotions. Expressive writing is a powerful tool to help you process difficult events. For details, see "Practice Expressive Writing" in Chapter 7, listed in *Practical Ways to Develop a Positive Mental Attitude.*

- **Immerse yourself in nature.** Being in nature can lead you to greater well-being and relaxation. A series of recent laboratory studies suggested that people who viewed nature scenes indoors and who reported being highly immersed in nature also reported higher valuing of intrinsic aspirations. Intrinsic aspirations (goals) are those that are inherently satisfying to pursue because they fulfill innate psychological needs for autonomy, relatedness, competence, and growth. You might expect that being in nature outdoors would elicit even stronger intrinsic aspirations and prosocial behaviors. Being in nature might elicit these aspirations by increasing connectedness with nature and increasing autonomy. Lab studies suggest that regular immersion in nature might also promote purposeful, other-oriented behaviors, such as volunteering[42].

- **Continue to work full- or part-time.** If you love your job and if it provides you with a sense of purpose and meaning in life, consider continuing to work instead of retiring at age 65. If full-time work is more than you want, how about part-time employment or contract work? The extra income might allow you to boost your charitable giving, thereby providing another source of purposeful activity.

- **Spend disposable income in prosocial ways.** If you have not already done so, identify a nonprofit organization whose mission especially resonates with you. Contribute a portion of your disposable income to that organization each year or, ideally, more frequently. Research indicates that prosocial spending leads to greater happiness than spending on tangible items, such as expensive consumer goods. The intentional activity of writing a check to your favorite nonprofit organization may motivate you to contribute your time to a worthy cause, thereby producing lasting happiness[43].

Three Key Points

1. *Live with Purpose* helps create meaning in life.

2. *Live with Purpose* promotes numerous aspects of vibrant health and emotional well-being.

3. Volunteering is a great way to *Live with Purpose*.

Chapter 9

Participate in a Spiritual Community

Substantial empirical evidence points to links between spiritual/religious factors and health in U.S. populations.
— William R. Miller

The healthy choice of participating in a spiritual community includes two facets. One is the value of belonging to and participating in a community whose values—especially those that support health and well-being—largely reflect our own. Being a member of a group of more or less like-minded people can help us make healthy choices and take action. The second facet is spiritual, which includes communities and groups of people who attempt to manifest daily, in thought and deed, their Higher Selves in the world.

"Religion" and "spirituality" are often used interchangeably in the scientific and medical literature, though many Americans identify as spiritual but not religious. Harold Koenig at Duke University writes extensively about the intersection of medicine, religion, spirituality, and health. Koenig distinguishes between religion and spirituality. He defines religion as a system of beliefs and practices observed by a community and supported by rituals that acknowledge, worship, and communicate with or approach the divine. He defines spirituality as a personal relationship with the transcendent. Koenig also notes that love, awe, forgiveness, gratitude, and support, all of which promote health and well-being, are not spirituality itself but arise from devoutly practiced spirituality.

Religion and Spirituality

In a recent report, Carolyn Aldwin at Oregon State University and her colleagues ascribed some health-related effects to religiousness and others to spirituality. Aldwin and colleagues defined religion as "the search for significance that occurs within the context of established institutions that are designed to facilitate spirituality." They defined spirituality as the search for the sacred and other aspects of life that are perceived to be manifestations of the divine, or imbued with divine-like qualities, such as transcendence. Aldwin and colleagues proposed a model in which religiousness mediates health through the self-regulation of healthy habits. Research shows that religiousness is associated with better health behaviors, including less smoking, lower alcohol consumption, and greater use of medical screenings. On the other hand, spirituality influences health primarily through the emotional regulation of physiological processes, including the body's major stress response system and its effects on inflammation. Measures of spirituality, as opposed to religiousness, are more strongly associated with biomarkers, such as blood pressure, cardiac reactivity, immune factors, and disease progression.

Aldwin and colleagues propose that both religion and spirituality affect social support, which promotes both behavioral and emotional self-regulation. If their model is valid, it suggests that interventions to foster healthy choices, including social support and beliefs about the importance of caring for the body, would be effective if people would draw upon their religious lives. Attempts to improve physiological health might be effective by helping people cultivate a richer spiritual life and, thereby, find the motivation to make healthy choices[1].

Benefits Linked to *Participate in a Spiritual Community*

The number of studies concerning religion, spirituality, and health began to skyrocket around the year 2000. Starting in mid-2010, Harold Koenig and his colleagues searched the literature for quantitative studies relating religion and/or spirituality to health. The terms "religion" and "spirituality" (R/S) were used interchangeably. Their search yielded 3,300 studies, with 2,100 of them dated 2000 or later. The studies were rated for methodological quality on a 10-point scale, with 10 being the highest. About 80 percent of those studies related to mental as opposed to physical health. Studies of mental health were sorted into ten categories: coping with adversity, positive emotions, depression, suicide, anxiety, schizophrenia, psychotic disorder, bipolar disorder, substance abuse, and social problems. For coping with adversity, the overwhelming majority of the studies showed that R/S was helpful[2].

Koenig further separated the positive emotions category into seven subcategories. For each subcategory, the percentages of studies that positively and significantly linked greater R/S with aspects of health were as follows: well-being/happiness (79 percent), hope (73 percent), optimism (81 percent), meaning and purpose (93 percent), self-esteem (61 percent), sense of control (61 percent), and positive character traits (70 percent). Studies that negatively and significantly linked R/S with health in any subcategory did not exceed eight percent; the link was usually near zero.

For depression, 61 percent of the studies reported a significant association between greater R/S and lower risk of depression. For suicide, anxiety, schizophrenia, substance abuse, and bipolar disorder, greater R/S was linked with lower risk for 75, 49, 33, 86, and 50 percent of the studies, respectively (but the last reflected only two studies). Less substance abuse was clearly related to greater R/S.

The researchers subdivided the social problems category into four subcategories. The percentages of studies that significantly linked greater R/S with lower risks negative aspects of health were as follows: delinquency/crime (79 percent) and marital instability (86 percent). The percentages of studies that significantly linked greater R/S to positive aspects of health were social support (82 percent) and social capital (79 percent).

R/S might positively affect mental health in three ways: (1) R/S could provide resources for improved coping with stress; (2) R/S could reduce stressful life experiences by promoting positive emotions and reducing negative ones through adherence to rules associated with R/S; and (3) R/S could promote prosocial behaviors that could reduce stress and increase social support.

Koenig identified five categories of health behaviors related to R/S. The percentages of studies that significantly and positively linked R/S with positive health behaviors were as follows: no cigarette smoking (90 percent), regular exercise (68 percent), healthy diet (62 percent), and lack of risky sexual behavior (86 percent). Curiously, greater R/S was statistically and positively linked to greater body weight.

Under the heading of R/S and physical health, Koenig identified 11 categories. The percentages of studies that significantly linked greater R/S to aspects physical health in a healthy direction were as follows: coronary heart disease (63 percent), hypertension (57 percent), cerebrovascular disease (44 percent, but with only nine studies), cerebrovascular disease (44 percent), Alzheimer's disease and dementia (48 percent), immune function (56 percent), endocrine function (74 percent), cancer (55 percent), physical functioning (36 percent), self-rated health (58 percent), pain and somatic symptoms (39 percent), and premature mortality (68 percent). Thus, greater R/S was linked to numerous important aspects of physical health.

Koenig offered several reasons why R/S might promote better physical health. R/S could improve psychological health that could lead to better physical health. R/S could promote better social relationships and sense of life purpose, leading to better access of health information and better health maintenance. R/S promotes better health behaviors, including less smoking, less alcohol and substance abuse, and better diet and more exercise, all of which lead to better physical health. Koenig emphasized that his research does not hinge on the existence of supernatural or transcendent forces, but in the belief that such forces exist. While R/S, in some instances, predicts adverse health consequences (such as higher body weight), Koenig's research overwhelmingly showed that R/S likely predicts better health behaviors and better mental and physical health[2].

According to Douglas Holtz-Eakin, the former director of the U.S. Congressional Budget Office, rising health care costs represent the central domestic issue of our time. Demographic, cultural, and financial factors, according to Holtz-Eakin, are coalescing to create a "perfect storm" in health care environments in the U.S. and other countries. Informal health ministries in religious communities will become more frequent and more relied upon in the decades ahead. The first responsibility for such ministries will be to promote healthy lifestyles—including diet and exercise—among members, and to conduct disease screenings. Koenig cites the Seventh Day Adventist, Lutheran Health Advocate Health Care, and Catholic Ascension Health Care systems as particularly active in this regard. The same is true for Mennonite and Brethren health care systems.

The studies highlighted in the rest of this chapter provide additional evidence for the broad range of health benefits linked to *Participate in a Spiritual Community*.

	Reduced risk of premature death
	Improved coping with stress
	Reduced risk of hypertension and lower blood pressure
Benefits Linked to	Increased well-being
Participate in a	Improved physical and mental health and health behaviors
Spiritual Community	Reduced risk of suicide
	Increased likelihood of making healthy choices
	Slower progression of HIV-AIDS
	Reduced allostatic load and lower risk of premature death

Reduced risk of premature death

Little doubt exists that religious involvement can help us cope with psychological and social stresses caused by heart disease, metabolic diseases, cognitive challenges with aging, and cancer. These chronic conditions can lead to chronic stress and negative emotions. Thus, curbing chronic stress and negative emotions may be a pathway by which religious involvement improves physical health. The effect of religious attendance on lowering mortality appears to be comparable to that of well-known factors such as cholesterol-lowering drugs, regular exercise, and smoking cessation. Religious attendance may therefore have a substantial public health impact, given that a 2017 Gallup Organization survey found that 37 percent of Americans reported being highly religious[3].

The Alameda County Study in California offered an opportunity to address the long-term relationships between religious attendance and mortality, as well as measures of health. The study began in 1965 with data collection on 6,928 persons (ages 16–94) who were followed until death or the year 1994, whichever came first. Compared to those with infrequent attendance in religious services, frequent (at least weekly) attendance predicted a significantly lower risk of premature death. The risk declined more for frequent attendees (predominantly women). Much of the salutary effect of religious attendance appeared to operate indirectly through better health behaviors. For instance, compared to participants who attended less than once a week or not at all, those who attended religious services at least weekly were *90 percent more likely to stop smoking*, plus 38 percent more likely to exercise more[4].

Frequent religious attendance (at least once weekly) was significantly positively associated with improved health practices, more stable marriages, and increased social connections for both men and women. Other possible explanations for improved health practices include peer influence, greater self-esteem, greater sense of control, proscribed unhealthy practices, increased value of social connection, and a tendency to treat one's body with respect[4].

A subsequent study drew from a much older population in the southeastern U.S. rather than the West Coast. Beginning in 1986, adults over age 65 living in four counties of central North Carolina were enrolled. Data on religious attendance and other health-related behaviors were available for 3,968 individuals. Participants who reported attending a religious service at least once a week were physically healthier, had more social support, and had healthier lifestyles than those who reported infrequent religious service attendance. After adjusting for a number of potentially confounding variables, the risk of dying prematurely for frequent religious service attendees over the six-year follow-up was 38 percent lower than for infrequent attenders. Therefore, people who regularly attended religious services appeared to receive one or more health benefits, apart from indirect benefits controlled for in the analysis. Frequent attenders of religious services likely benefit from greater social support and healthier lifestyle choices, including lower cigarette and alcohol consumption[5].

A paper published in 2000 represented the first meta-analysis of data from 29 previously published studies to quantitatively address R/S and mortality. Across these studies, very religious individuals had 29 percent higher odds of survival during the respective follow-up periods than less religious individuals. Analysis of the variables suggested that the positive association of religion and survival arose from public rather than private religious activity. The impact of the religious effect on mortality was small but similar to that for psychosocial factors. The association of religious involvement and mortality was robust, in that the association occurred regardless of the length of the follow-up period. Based on this meta-analysis alone, little doubt exists that greater religious involvement predicts lower risk of premature death[6].

Researchers at Harvard confirmed the statistically significant associations between religious attendance and mortality found in previous longitudinal studies. The study used data from 74,536 women in the Nurses' Health Study, which began in 1976 and enrolled 121,700 female nurses ages 30–55. Among the subjects, religious attendance was categorized as either more than once a week, once a week, 1–3 times per month, less than once per month, or never/almost never. Compared to women who never attended religious services, those who attended more than once a week had a 33 percent lower risk of all-cause death over the 16-year follow-up period. The comparable reduced risks of death from cardiovascular disease and all types of cancer were 27 and 21 percent, respectively. The results were robust across different racial and ethnic groups and across the follow-up period. The size of the effect of religious attendance on the risk of premature death was comparable to that of other health behaviors. Depressive symptoms, smoking, social support, and optimism mediated the effect of religious attendance on the risk of mortality, with social support and smoking having the greatest impact[7].

While accumulating research links R/S to reduced risk of premature death, the mechanisms that might bolster this link remain uncertain. A new study used data from 5,200 participants in the Health and Retirement Study to test a variety of possible mediators that could affect mortality. Researchers found 10 variables that significantly affected the relationship between R/S and mortality risk. Variables linked to lower risk of premature death included greater life satisfaction, weekly (or more) contact with friends, more exercise, fewer physical functioning problems, and less hopelessness and anger. Depressive symptoms, anxiety, and excessive alcohol consumption were associated with an increased risk of premature death. While the magnitudes of the mediators were individually small, their collective impact on mortality risk could be substantial[8].

Researchers at Harvard used data from 36,313 participants in the Black Women's Health Study from 2005 to 2010 to look at other measures of religion or spirituality on longevity. Results showed that religious coping and self-described religiosity or spirituality may reduce the risk of death indirectly through health-related behaviors such as not smoking, consuming minimal alcohol, and increasing physical activity. However, church attendance appeared to have the strongest direct effect on African American women for extending their longevity. Frequency of prayer not was linked to risk of premature death[9].

Improved coping with stress

People under chronic stress often exhibit poor health habits that can affect physical health and functioning. Psychological and social stresses negatively affect immune, endocrine, and cardiovascular functions. These adverse physiological changes can increase our body's susceptibility to metabolic, neurologic, cardiac, and circulatory diseases. On the other hand, positive social interactions and emotional states can boost immune, endocrine, and cardiovascular functions, thereby protecting against disease or slowing its progression. If religious or spiritual involvement enhances psychological health and social interactions, it follows that religious or spiritual factors may improve physical health, too. The pathways could include reducing psychological stress, increasing social support, and encouraging positive health behaviors. Participating in a spiritual community might promote health in three ways: (1) as a coping strategy that helps defuse chronic stress; (2) as a prosocial force that promotes volunteering and other altruistic behaviors, which could help create a purposeful life; and (3) as a method of behavioral control that encourages healthy choices and habit formation[10].

Psychologist Crystal Park proposed a meaning-making model to account for the observed relationships between people's meaning in life and their health and well-being. The model assumes that differences between persons' situational meaning and their global meaning create distress. In turn, psychic discomfort spurs efforts to reduce the difference and, therefore, the distress. In this context, global meaning includes beliefs, goals, and a sense of purpose. In situations where people have little opportunity to directly alter their circumstances, meaning making involves effortful coping to change their appraisal of a situation or their global meaning. Global beliefs can promote personal health through an increased sense of control, goal setting, and a greater sense that life has meaning. Meaning making can help persons with chronic conditions cope better by reappraising their conditions. For example, a person could reappraise a cancer diagnosis from a catastrophe to an opportunity for personal growth and development. Therefore, spirituality may foster stress-related personal growth by helping people both find meaning in challenging circumstances and to cope resourcefully[11].

Reduced risk of hypertension and lower blood pressure

Does attendance at religious services predict a reduced risk of hypertension and lower blood pressure? Researchers collected data from the National Health and Nutrition Examination Survey III, a nationally representative sample of 14,475 Americans over age 20 at baseline, to find out. After adjusting for confounding factors, participants attending religious services at least weekly were 24 percent less likely to have hypertension (a systolic blood pressure of 140 mm Hg or greater or a diastolic blood pressure of 90 mm Hg or greater) and had a significantly lower systolic blood pressure than those who never attended religious services. Systolic blood pressure declined as religious service attendance increased from zero to 1–51 times per year, 52 times per year, and more than 52 times per year[12].

Increased well-being

Subjective well-being can rise after a particularly delightful life event, but it typically falls back in a few months. Alas, a negative event is more likely than a positive event to create a long-lasting effect. Researchers devised two studies to determine: (1) if well-being increased following attendance at religious services or physical exercise, and (2) if well-being increased even more as the frequency of attendance in religious services increased. Subjects for the first study included 2,095 attendees at 37 churches in the Boston area. Subjects for the second study included 224 patrons at a gym and two yoga classes. In both studies, one group of people was interviewed entering the religious service or exercise session and a different group was interviewed exiting it. Subjective well-being was evaluated as the composite of answers to three questions. As expected, subjects reported significantly greater well-being after the religious service or exercise session compared to before it. Furthermore, the increase was greater for persons who attended more services or exercise sessions during the previous month. Therefore, increased well-being may arise from frequent, regular, relatively short religious services or exercise sessions[13].

As noted earlier, Harold Koenig[2] summarized approximately 3,300 studies published before 2010 that evaluated connections between R/S and various aspects of positive mental health, negative mental health, health behaviors, and physical health. Koenig's review of research published after 2010 confirmed his earlier results[14]. Thus, there appears to be little doubt that persons who *Participate in a Spiritual Community* are more likely than those who don't to possess greater well-being and greater meaning and purpose in life. These benefits might arise from more exercise, a better diet, and less smoking, less alcohol consumption, and less depression, among other possibilities.

Reduced risk of suicide

Past studies have linked participation in religious services to a reduced suicide risk. However, many of these studies suffered from methodological problems. A long-term study that controlled for depression at baseline avoided those deficiencies. Researchers used data for 89,708 participants (women only) in the Nurses' Health Study who were followed from 1992 to 1996. During that period, 36 suicides were recorded. The relative risk of suicide for women who attended weekly or more frequent religious services was 85 percent lower than the risk for women who never attended. The differences were even more striking for Catholic women attending weekly services, whose risk of suicide was 95 percent lower. Overall, the suicide rate for all female nurses was about half that for the general U.S. population. More social integration, fewer depressive symptoms, and lower alcohol consumption partially explained the association between religious service attendance and lower suicide risk for infrequent but not for frequent attenders. The fact that the major religious traditions hold that suicide is morally wrong might help explain these findings[15].

Increased likelihood of making healthy choices

The Alameda County Study mentioned earlier in this chapter prompted researchers to explore ways in which religious attendance could improve longevity, perhaps by making and maintaining healthy choices. A follow-up study by William Strawbridge and colleagues[16] addressed this, using data from 2,676 participants who enrolled in the original Alameda County Study in 1965 and survived to 1994. Participants (women and men combined) who reported frequent (at least weekly) religious attendance in 1965 had a greater likelihood of making healthy choices over the subsequent 30 years than participants who attended church services less frequently or not at all. More specifically, from the 1965 baseline, the odds of quitting smoking and becoming more physically active were 78 and 54 percent higher, respectively, for frequent religious service attendees compared to less-than-weekly or non-attendees. Similarly, the odds of recovering from being depressed, increasing the number of individual social relationships, and getting—and staying—married were 131, 62, and 57 percent higher, respectively, for frequent religious service attendees. Notably, people attending religious services frequently did not begin the study having already made healthy choices. The effects of religious attendance were more pronounced for women than men. Frequent religious service attenders attendees exhibited a lower likelihood of making poor health-related choices. For example, frequent attenders had a 28 percent lower risk of skipping annual physical check-ups, a 37 percent lower risk of reducing social relationships, and a 49 percent lower risk of becoming divorced or separated compared to those who attended religious services less frequently or not at all. Again, effects were stronger for women than men. These findings align with previous research that found women in general have a stronger religious commitment than men, and more likely than men to use religion as a means to cope with stressful events. Participants in a spiritual community may make better health-related choices and can enjoy greater longevity as a consequence.

Slower progression of HIV-AIDS

Some people become more religious or spiritual after experiencing a traumatic event. A diagnosis of HIV-AIDS would be a traumatic event for most of us. Researchers at the University of Miami wanted to know if people receiving such a diagnosis become more religious or spiritual and, if so, whether the course of their disease changed. The study's subjects included 100 people with HIV-AIDS, many of whom were poor. At baseline, the subjects filled out questionnaires that evaluated health behaviors, depression, optimism, and social support. Three years into the study, R/S was evaluated with five questions. Results showed that 45 percent of the subjects became more religious or spiritual, 42 percent remained the same, and 13 percent became less religious or spiritual, after controlling for church attendance. The loss of a key type of white blood cell (CD4) was 4.5 times faster in those who showed decreased religiousness or spirituality. Viral load increased more slowly in those who experienced an increase in religiousness or spirituality after diagnosis. People who became more religious or spiritual after receiving an HIV-AIDS diagnosis had a significantly slower progression of the disease[17].

Reduced allostatic load and lower risk of premature death

Stress reduction provides a mechanism by which attending religious services could promote better health. Researchers used data from the National Health and Nutrition Examination Survey III to determine whether allostatic load affected the link between religiosity and risk of premature death. Allostatic load reflects the physiological effects of repeated or chronic challenges the body experiences as stressful. Allostatic load was evaluated based on levels of 10 clinical biomarkers, such as systolic blood pressure. Over an average follow-up of 14 years and compared to participants who attended church at least once per year, those who did not attend church had a 24 and 38 percent higher risk of exhibiting a medium and high allostatic load, respectively. Compared with non–churchgoers, churchgoers had a significantly lower risk of premature death. The risk of premature death decreased as the frequency of church attendance increased from less than weekly to weekly to more than weekly, even after adjusting for confounding factors[18].

Poor Outcomes Linked to Failing to *Participate in a Spiritual Community*

The previous eight chapters each included a section on poor health and well-being outcomes associated with failing to follow the respective healthy lifestyle choices. This chapter is different. Studies that show positive effects of religious/spirituality could be interpreted as suggesting that the lack of participation in a spiritual community would lead to poor outcomes. Yet studies that directly address the idea that people who fail to *Participate in a Spiritual Community* suffer poor health-related outcomes appear to be sparse. Here are several examples.

The Centers for Disease Control and Prevention used data from 11,820 adult participants in the National Health and Nutrition Examination Survey III to determine if frequency of attendance at religious services was associated with leisure-time physical activity. Frequent attendees were those who reported attending 52 or more times per year. Infrequent attendees were those who reported attending church fewer than 52 times annually. Leisure-time daily physical activities included walking, cycling, gardening, and trips to the gym. For women frequent attendees aged 60 or older and without mobility limitation, infrequent attendees had a 40 percent higher chance of reporting no leisure-time physical activity. No significant associations occurred for younger women or men of any age[19].

A review of the literature examining the impact of spirituality on mental health concluded that "other aspects of spirituality seem to have no effect on mental health or, in some cases, can lead to feelings of guilt, shame or powerlessness, which can be damaging or harmful to a person's mental health"[20].

In a study that used data from the 1996 Genera Social Survey, Ellison and colleagues found that strong beliefs in the pervasiveness of sin were strongly linked with anxiety[21], while in 2011 Reeves and colleagues argued that religious beliefs may provoke delusions in some psychiatric patients[22]. Overall, however, the upside benefits of participating in a spiritual community appear to vastly exceed the downside risks.

Meeting Patients' Spiritual Needs

Participating in a spiritual community predicts positive health outcomes, such as increased longevity, reduced risk of suicide by U.S. women, and greater social support/assistance while recovering from major illness. These benefits might arise directly from making healthy lifestyle choices, or indirectly from better social integration and social support, developing an optimistic attitude, and living with purpose. In any event, the medical establishment tends to give spirituality short shrift, even for patients who express a desire for spiritual support during medical care. A telling example: One hundred patients with advanced lung cancer ranked faith in God as the *second most important factor* (out of seven total) in medical decision making, while physicians ranked it last[23].

Religious beliefs frequently affect the kind of health care a person wants to receive. These beliefs affect how a person copes with illness, finds purpose, and derives meaning when feeling physical pain or being unable to complete previously simple tasks. Such beliefs, which help us maintain hope and motivation toward self-care when our lives are in turmoil, presumably also lead to better health. Nevertheless, few physicians inquire about the spiritual needs of their patients or are even open to doing so. Consequently, if we end up in the hospital or in hospice, we may need to be assertive in discussing our spiritual needs with the resident medical staff and our doctor.

> *"More explicit focus on spirituality, often considered outside the realm of modern medicine, could improve person-centered approaches to well-being long sought by patients and clinicians."*
> – T. J. VanderWeele, Tracy A. Balboni, and Howard K. Hoh[24]

Practical Ways to *Participate in a Spiritual Community*

- **Attend social events.** Churches and spiritual centers typically sponsor social events such as potlucks and trips to interesting places. Costs are typically low, and events offer a wonderful opportunity to make new friends.

- **Attend classes.** Churches and spiritual groups almost always offer classes. The church I attend has ongoing classes, such as grief support, and one-time events, often led by outside speakers.

- **Volunteer.** Churches and spiritual groups rely on volunteer labor. Serving as an usher for weekly services, maintaining the church building and grounds, answering the phone, stuffing envelopes, or working in the church kitchen will also help *Cultivate Social Connections*.

Three Key Points

1. Participating in a spiritual community both directly and indirectly supports numerous aspects of health and well-being.

2. The health benefits of participating in a spiritual community do not necessarily arise from the existence of a supernatural being or transcendent forces but in the belief that it/they exist.

3. The positive effects of the healthy choice *Participate in a Spiritual Community* appear to arise largely from making other healthy choices, including *Cultivate Social Connections* and *Defuse Chronic Stress*.

Chapter 10

The Benefits of Multiple Healthy Lifestyle Choices

Exercise, social connection, and optimism all tie for first place in terms of keeping your brain healthy.
— Andrew Newberg and Mark Robert Waldman[1]

U p to this point, we've considered healthy lifestyle choices as if they were independent of one another. But that's not how life really works. Our lifestyle choices act in concert to produce the level of health and well-being that we experience. Yet relatively few published studies take into account multiple healthy lifestyle choices, largely due to cost and logistical complexity. Nevertheless, some studies do illustrate the power of adopting multiple healthy choices to foster long-term health and well-being. As you read this chapter, you'll notice that the vast majority of healthy choices (or the opposite—risk factors) apply mostly to the physical body. That imbalance reflects the available scientific and medical literature rather than a lack of efficacy of other healthy choices that affect primarily the mind or spirit.

Lifestyle Choices and Behaviors Most Associated with Better Health

In 1965, a group of researchers initiated a longitudinal study to understand possible relationships between personal health habits, quality of life, and mortality. A representative sample of 6,928 people living in Alameda County, California, just north of Berkeley, formed the cohort. Initially, the study focused on seven healthy lifestyle choices, dubbed the Alameda 7, that researchers thought might be associated with better health and greater longevity: (1) sleeping seven to eight hours per night, (2) eating breakfast, (3) eating between meals, (4) maintaining a healthy weight, (5) getting regular exercise, (6) limiting alcohol consumption, and (7) not smoking. Subsequent research showed that five of the initial seven—sleeping seven to eight hours per night, maintaining a healthy weight, getting regular exercise, limiting alcohol consumption, and not smoking—were strongly associated with various measures of health and longevity. Additional research on the Alameda County cohort showed that social and marital relationships, religiosity, and sleep disturbances also predicted better personal health. The Alameda County research alerted the medical and public health communities to the likelihood that our daily choices and the habits that arise from them substantially affect our health and well-being[2].

A more recent study evaluated the impact of 10 modifiable daily behaviors on long-term outcomes for a diverse adult working population. A group of 10,248 participants enrolled during 2003 in a voluntary workplace wellness program at Vanderbilt University. The participants were followed for nine years. A low-fat diet, aerobic exercise, not smoking, and getting adequate sleep were the behaviors most significantly associated with future positive health outcomes. A dose-response relationship occurred between dietary fat intake levels and the tendency to develop hypertension, obesity, diabetes, heart disease, and/or high cholesterol. After dietary fat, aerobic exercise was the next most significant behavior associated with influencing health outcomes. Compared with sedentary participants, those who exercised four days per week experienced the following reductions in risk: new-onset diabetes (69 percent), heart disease (54 percent), and high cholesterol (39 percent). A low-fat diet and adequate sleep were more beneficial than some commonly promoted healthy behaviors, such as eating breakfast. Based on this study, top priorities for workplace health promotion would include adopting a low-fat diet, aerobic exercise, not smoking, and adequate sleep[3].

Benefits Linked to Multiple Healthy Lifestyle Choices

There is no doubt that lifestyle choices affect health-related outcomes. But according to the research and writings of Roger Walsh at the University of California, Irvine, health professionals have significantly underestimated the importance of lifestyle on mental health. Walsh identifies exercise, nutrition, time in nature, relationships, recreation, stress management, religious/spiritual involvement, and contributions and service to others as key factors to maintaining positive mental health. (These should sound familiar by now!) Exercise compares favorably to medication as a therapy for depression. Additionally, Walsh notes that while health professionals themselves exercise, only 10 percent of health professionals recommend exercise to their patients.

Summarizing a literature review on the effects and effectiveness of various lifestyle changes, Walsh writes that recommended foods include fish, vegetables, and probably fruit, with animal fats de-emphasized. Recreation and contemplation in natural settings can enhance both physical and mental health, including greater cognitive, attentional, emotional, and spiritual subjective well-being—and increase stress management skills. Good relationships with other people predict greater happiness, quality of life, resilience, and cognitive capacity. However, in the digital age, with electronic gadgets connecting us virtually, the number of human relationships and their intimacy seem to be declining. Walsh notes that service to others can provide more benefit to the giver than the receiver, including greater purpose in life, while religious/spiritual involvement can foster service and contributions to others, greater life purpose, and better health behaviors[4].

Sadly, many people have little social support and/or don't understand the power of healthy lifestyle choices. Such people may believe that healing arises from an outside authority or from medication, as opposed to their daily lifestyle choices. Unfortunately, doctors often fail to promote healthy lifestyle choices to their patients or do so ineffectively. Walsh argues that given the medical care costs associated with a typical American lifestyle, embracing healthier choices needs to be a centerpiece of personal and public health initiatives. This chapter makes the case that we are likely to enjoy huge benefits from making multiple healthy lifestyle choices.

Benefits Linked to Multiple Healthy Lifestyle Choices

- Increased *Quality of Lifespan*
- Increased longevity
- Lower risk of sudden cardiac death
- Reduced risk of cardiovascular disease
- Reduced risk of coronary heart disease
- Improved cardiac rehabilitation
- Improved coronary risk factors
- Reduced risk of stroke
- Reduced risk of dementia
- Reduced risk of chronic disease
- Increased cognitive function
- Reduced risk of type 2 diabetes
- Reduced risk of colorectal cancer
- Maintaining mobility in old age

Increased *Quality of Lifespan*

To assess whether embracing healthy lifestyle choices in midlife can increase *Quality of Lifespan*—namely, greater longevity without disability—researchers used data from the Honolulu Heart Program and the Honolulu Asia Aging Study to find out. A total of 5,820 men of Japanese American ancestry, free of illness and functional impairments, and with an average age of 54 years, were followed for up to 40 years (1965–2005). For each subject, researchers evaluated nine risk factors: overweight, high blood glucose, high triglycerides, hypertension, low grip strength, ever being a smoker, high alcohol consumption, low education, and being unmarried. All these factors can be modified by healthy lifestyle choices. **The probability of these men surviving to age 85—with no chronic illness, cognitive or physical impairment—was 55 percent if they had none of the nine modifiable risk factors, compared to 9 percent for men with six or more of the risk factors—a six-fold difference!** Making healthy lifestyle choices may greatly increase our *Quality of Lifespan*[5].

Authorities recommend limiting alcohol consumption to one standard drink per day for women and two for men. A standard alcoholic drink in the U.S. has about 14 grams of alcohol. One 12-ounce can of beer, one five-ounce glass of wine, and one mixed drink with 1.5 ounces of spirits contains that amount of alcohol.

Studies on identical twins show that genes account for only about 25 percent of the variation in longevity, with lifestyle choices and other factors accounting for the remaining 75 percent. In other words, lifestyle choices can substantially improve survival for men and women. In fact, the benefits of making multiple healthy lifestyle choices—including greater longevity, overall health, and functionality in life—also apply to older people. The Physician's Health Study began with 22,071 male physicians (average age 72 years) who enrolled between 1981 and 1984. A subgroup included 2,357 men who were born on or before December 31, 1915. These subgroup participants had the potential to survive to age 90 until March 31, 2006, when the study stopped. At baseline, the participants were apparently healthy with no history of cardiovascular disease, cancer, or other major diseases. Over 25 years of follow-up, 970 survived to or beyond age 90, and 1,387 died. Participants who were overweight, hypertensive, diabetic, and smokers had a significantly higher risk of dying compared to participants of normal body weight, who had neither hypertension nor diabetes, and who never smoked. The incidence of cancer and cardiovascular disease was lower among participants who survived to the end of the study (March 31, 2006) compared to participants who died before the end of the study. Cancer and cardiovascular disease occurred from three to five years later for the healthier participants. Regular exercise was associated with a 30 percent increased likelihood of survival over 25 years. **Participants who exhibited the positive effects of healthy choices (body-mass index less than 30, never smoked, normal blood pressure, no diabetes, exercised at moderate intensity two to four times per week) at age 70 had a 54 percent chance of surviving until age 90. Participants who exhibited none of these positive effects had a mere 4 percent chance.** Men who survived to age 90 had significantly better physical function and mental well-being, less depression, and better self-reported health than men who died during follow-up. These results support an earlier hypothesis that people who adopt healthy choices can live longer, avoid or postpone illness and injury, and live better during their longer life than people who don't adopt healthy choices. Older men who adopt healthy choices can expect to improve their *Quality of Lifespan*[6].

Increased longevity

While the longevity benefits of individual healthy choices are well documented, their combined effects are less well documented. Data from the European Prospective Investigation into Cancer and Nutrition provided an opportunity to evaluate the individual and combined effects of healthy choices. Between 1993 and 1997, 20,244 men and women aged 45–79 were recruited from Norfolk County in the United Kingdom. Researchers identified four health-related behaviors: (1) not smoking, (2) high fruit and high vegetable consumption, (3) limited alcohol consumption, and (4) some level of physical activity. After an average of 11 years of follow-up, all four health factors significantly predicted all-cause mortality. Smoking was the most consistent and strongest risk factor. **Participants with zero healthy behaviors had a three-fold higher risk of dying over the 11-year follow-up period than participants with four healthy behaviors.** For death from cardiovascular disease and cancer, the comparable relative risks were four-fold and nearly three-fold higher, respectively. When segregated by sex for all-cause mortality, men and women with zero healthy behaviors had a 3.11-fold and 4.23-fold higher relative risk of dying, respectively. **The mortality risk of participants with four healthy choices was equivalent to living 14 years longer in chronological age.** Multiple healthy lifestyle choices strongly predicted much lower risk of premature death in this sample of U.K. residents[7].

A meta-analysis of 15 longitudinal studies investigated the extent to which multiple healthy lifestyle factors are associated with the risk of dying during the respective follow-up periods. The average follow-up was 13 years. Healthy lifestyle criteria included the following: (1) never smoked; (2) optimal body weight (BMI between 18.5 and 25.0); (3) physically active (more than 3.5 hours per week); (4) healthy diet (in the upper 20 percent of a healthy diet score); and (5) moderate alcohol consumption (5–15 grams per day for women or 5–30 grams per day for men). **The risk of dying during follow-up declined with each additional lifestyle factor used in the data analysis: from 0.72 for one factor, 0.58 for two factors, 0.46 for three factors, and 0.34 for four factors. Thus, a person with four healthy lifestyle factors would enjoy a 66 percent lower risk of death during follow-up compared to a person with zero healthy lifestyle factors. The authors commented that the number of healthy lifestyle factors adopted might be more important than which factors they might be.** This study provides convincing evidence that our longevity increases as the number of healthy lifestyles we embrace increases[8].

Lower risk of sudden cardiac death

To understand how combined lifestyle choices might impact the risk of sudden cardiac death, one report used data from 81,722 subjects from the Nurses' Health Study (NHS). This long-term study began in 1984, with follow-up until 2010. A low-risk lifestyle included four factors: (1) not smoking, (2) a body-mass index less than 25, (3) more than 30 minutes of exercise per day, and (4) ranked in the top 40 percent of the alternate Mediterranean diet score. The alternate Mediterranean diet emphasizes a high intake of vegetables, fruits, nuts, legumes, whole grains, fish, and moderate alcohol. **Women with a low-risk lifestyle had a 92 percent lower risk for sudden cardiac death compared to women with no low-risk factors. If the association was causal, 81 percent of the sudden cardiac deaths could theoretically have been prevented if all the women had adhered to a low-risk lifestyle.** While 80 percent of women in the study didn't smoke, most women didn't embrace other healthful habits. Only eight percent of the women were at low risk of sudden cardiac death from all four lifestyle factors. On the bright side, there's a huge potential for improvement[9].

In another study, Swedish researchers set out to discover whether healthy lifestyle choices that confer protective effects on younger people could also confer protective effects on older people. In 1987, the researchers enrolled residents age 75 and older in the Kings-holmen district of central Stockholm. The cohort consisted of 1,810 participants who were followed until 2005. Participants were classified according to their risk for mortality with respect to four unhealthy lifestyle factors: (1) overweight or underweight, (2) current or former smoker, (3) limited or poor social network, and (4) lack of engagement in leisure-time activities. Compared to those who died during 18 years of follow-up, survivors were more likely to be women (as opposed to men); more highly educated; have healthy lifestyle factors (moderate weight, never a smoker, better social network, participation in more leisure-time activities); and have no chronic health conditions. **Compared to those in the high-risk group for mortality (based on four unhealthy lifestyle factors), the median survival for those in the low-risk group (with no unhealthy lifestyle factors) was 5.3 years longer for women and 6.3 years longer for men.** Evidently, healthy lifestyle choices can improve longevity for both younger and older people. Thus, it's never too late to adopt healthy choices and turn them into healthy habits[10].

Reduced risk of cardiovascular disease

Harvard researchers used data from the NHS to study the risk of cardiovascular disease, including heart attacks and strokes. The researchers defined the low-risk women as those who: (1) never smoked; (2) had a body-mass index less than 25; (3) did moderate to vigorous exercise at least half an hour per day; (4) ate a diet rich in fiber, omega-3 fatty acids, and folic acid (enriched foods, dried beans, avocados, vegetables, seeds, nuts); and (5) consumed at least one-half of an alcoholic drink per day. **Compared to women who didn't adopt any low-risk lifestyle choices, those who adopted all five low-risk lifestyle choices reduced their risk of cardiovascular disease by 87 percent over the 14-year follow-up period.** However, only three percent of the women—nurses, mind you—landed in the low-risk category[11].

The lifetime risk of cardiovascular disease, despite being the leading cause of death in the U.S., was unknown until recently. The Framingham Heart Study provided data to address this point. Subjects included 3,564 men and 4,362 women at least 50 years of age and free of cardiovascular disease at baseline. The six factors evaluated in the study included total cholesterol, HDL cholesterol, systolic or diastolic blood pressure, diabetic status, smoking status, and body-mass index. **Men with no unhealthy factors had a lifetime risk of cardiovascular disease of 5 percent, while those with two or more unhealthy factors had a 69 percent risk. For women, the comparable risks were 8 percent and 50 percent. Men and women who had no unhealthy factors lived an average of 11 and 8 years longer, respectively, than men and women with two or more unhealthy factors.** This study shows that healthy lifestyle choices can pay huge dividends into our health and longevity accounts[12].

Healthy Choices Improve Biomarkers of Cardiovascular Disease

Adopting multiple healthy choices might reduce our risk of cardiovascular disease by improving our physiology. To find out whether healthy choices would improve biomarkers of cardiovascular disease, researchers used data from the National Health and Nutrition Examination Survey, a nationally representative sample of U.S. adults. The four healthy lifestyle characteristics included getting 150 minutes per week of moderate-intensity physical activity, eating a healthy diet, not smoking, and 5-20 percent body fat (men) or 8-30 percent (women). **Compared to those participants with zero healthy lifestyle characteristics, individuals with three to four healthy lifestyle characteristics had more favorable levels in 10 out of 13 biomarkers.** (Exceptions were mean arterial blood pressure, fasting glucose, and HbA1c.) Being physically active was associated favorably with nine of the 13 biomarkers, while having a normal body fat percentage was associated favorably with 10 of the biomarkers. Therefore, *Keep Moving* and *Eat Better* can positively affect our physiology[13].

Reduced risk of coronary heart disease

Research has identified several healthy lifestyle choices that individually predict lower risk of developing coronary heart disease. But little is known about their *joint* effects on the risk of coronary heart disease ion middle-aged men, especially those taking drugs to reduce blood pressure or cholesterol. Researchers at Harvard used data from 42,847 men aged 40–75 years at baseline to address this shortcoming. The researchers defined healthy lifestyle choices as: (1) not currently smoking, (2) moderate body mass (BMI less than 25), (3) modest alcohol consumption (5–30 grams per day), (4) being physically active (more than 30 minutes per day of moderate-intensity or strenuous exercise), and (5) following a good diet (scoring in the top 40 percent of adherence to the Alternative Healthy Eating Index). **Over 16 years of follow-up, men who adopted all five healthy lifestyle choices had** an 87 percent lower risk of coronary heart disease compared to those who made no healthy choices. The risk declined in a progressive manner as the number of healthy habits increased from 1 to 5 for medication users and non-medication users alike. Extrapolating the trend of relative risk to six health habits showed zero relative risk of coronary heart disease. The health professionals in this study probably followed better health habits than Americans in general. Thus, the beneficial effects of adopting all five of these healthy choices would likely be even greater across the entire U.S. population. Yet, a mere four percent of the participants in the study exhibited all five healthy choices. There's lots of room for improvement[14].

Healthy Lifestyle Factors Protect Against Coronary Artery Disease

Calcification of coronary arteries increases the risk of coronary heart disease. The Multi-Ethnic Study of Atherosclerosis, which ran from 2000 to 2010, investigated which healthy lifestyle choices protect against coronary artery disease. Participants included 6,229 individuals between ages 44 and 84 at baseline who were recruited from around the U.S. Healthy lifestyle factors included (1) diet (median or greater adherence score for a Mediterranean diet), (2) body-mass index (between 18.5 and 24.9), (3) never smoking, and (4) regular physical activity (at least 150 minutes of moderate-intensity activity or at least 75 minutes of strenuous activity per week). **Participants with all four healthy lifestyle factors had an 81 percent lower risk of dying over the average follow-up of 7.6 years compared to those with no healthy factors.** In absolute terms, those with three or four healthy factors had a 4.9 percent risk of dying, while those with zero healthy factors had a 8.8 percent risk of dying during the follow-up period. The odds of developing coronary artery calcification over an average follow-up of 3.1 years was 46 percent lower for those with four healthy factors compared to those with none. **Interestingly, healthy lifestyle factors were a better predictor of premature death than was cardiovascular disease. This difference suggests that the benefits of healthy habits extend beyond the cardiovascular realm to other chronic diseases, perhaps including cancer.** Sadly, only two percent of all participants and less than one percent of black and Hispanic participants exhibited all four healthy factors[15].

Improved cardiac rehabilitation

In the 1990, cardiologist Dean Ornish and colleagues published a breakthrough study of an intensive cardiac rehabilitation program called the Lifestyle Heart Trial (LHT). Research with mostly men patients showed that the program yielded clinically significant improvements in risk factors for cardiovascular disease and in cardiovascular disease symptoms[16]. Because the clinical research was compelling, the LHT expanded to eight sites around the U.S. to find out whether it could be implemented successfully elsewhere, while including more women. Research subjects included 347 men and 93 women. Each patient was assigned to either group 1 or group 2. Group 1 included patients with diagnosed cardiovascular disease. Group 2 included patients with coronary artery bypass or angioplasty. The program featured a healthy diet, moderate exercise, social support, and stress management. Researchers encouraged participants to eat a low fat diet emphasizing fruits, vegetables, grains, legumes, nonfat dairy, and egg whites. Participants were also urged to get at least three hours per week of moderate-intensity exercise, such as brisk walking. Subjects were asked to attend group support meetings and to practice stress management activities, such as restorative yoga, for one hour per day. **Both men and women in the LHT program (featuring four healthy behaviors) showed significant improvement in diet, exercise, and stress management over one year. Moreover, both men and women showed small but significant improvements in body weight, blood pressure, heart rate, total cholesterol, and LDL cholesterol. Exercise capacity also increased along with physical functioning, reduced bodily pain, general health, vitality, social functioning, and mental health.** Most of the improvement occurred during the first three months of the program. Thus, participants did not have to wait long for improvements to manifest themselves. Improvements were more pronounced for women than men. This study demonstrated that the positive results of the LHT apply to a broader population[17].

The next step for Ornish and his colleagues was to test the LHT program at clinical/community sites across the U.S. A total of 2,974 men and women were recruited at sites in Illinois, Nebraska, Pennsylvania, and West Virginia for an intensive one-year cardiac rehab program. As before, the program centered on a healthy diet, moderate exercise, social support, and stress management. The recommended low-fat diet still included fruits, vegetables, whole grains, and legumes but with the addition of soy products and minimally refined carbohydrates. Participants were urged to get at least three hours per week of moderate-intensity exercise, such as brisk walking. They were also advised to attend group support meetings and to practice stress management activities, such as restorative yoga, for one hour per day. **From baseline to 12 weeks and continuing for one year, participants following the multipronged cardiac rehab program exhibited dramatic drops in hyperlipidemia (excess fats in the blood, from 79 to 20 percent); hypertension (from 74 to 19 percent); and obesity (from 68 to 17 percent). For those participants with**

complete data sets, all the measured factors—triglycerides; total, LDL, and HDL cholesterol; systolic and diastolic blood pressure; dietary fat; hemoglobin HbA1c; exercise; functional capacity; hostility; and depression—moved significantly in the healthful direction from baseline to 12 weeks (except for HDL cholesterol, which was unchanged). From 12 weeks to one year, most of the factors moved in the unhealthful direction, but at one year, levels of these factors were significantly better than at baseline. This research confirmed the effectiveness of the intensive cardiac rehab program based on four healthy choices and implemented at clinical and community sites across the U.S. Interestingly, the Ornish LHT program was one of the few that emphasized social support and stress management, which are two of the nine healthy lifestyle choices that this book champions[18].

Improved coronary risk factors

The Multisite Cardiac Lifestyle Intervention Program (MCLIP)—which introduced and evaluated several health behaviors in cardiac patients—reduced markers for coronary heart disease and reduced the number of clinical cardiac events in cardiac patients. A follow-up study sought to determine if low-socioeconomic-status patients in Illinois, Nebraska, Pennsylvania, and West Virginia would enjoy the same coronary heart disease benefits as patients of higher socioeconomic status. Education served as the primary indicator of socioeconomic status for 785 patients, with income as a secondary indicator because income data were available for only 478 patients. The study ran for three months, with two four-hour sessions each week. Each session typically featured a patient interaction with a nurse, interactive lectures, cooking demonstrations, one hour of supervised exercise, one hour of group support, and one hour of stress management. As in other MCLIP trials, participants were encouraged to eat a low-fat, low-protein, high-complex-carbohydrate diet. **At three months, the low- and high-socioeconomic-status participants showed similar attendance and adherence to the program's healthy interventions. Both groups also showed significant improvement in coronary risk factors, including body weight, blood pressure, total and LDL cholesterol, triglycerides, HbA1c, depression, perceived stress, hostility, and quality of life. Reduction in dietary fat and improvements in exercise amount, exercise capacity, and stress management were higher for participants in the low-socioeconomic group.** This study found that the low-socioeconomic group of coronary heart disease patients benefited significantly from the MCLIP[19]. Would such an effective program someday be covered by universal health insurance for Americans?

Reduced risk of stroke

Long-term studies show significant associations between clusters of lifestyle choices and reduced risk of coronary heart disease. Given that certain types of strokes arise from defects in the circulatory system, it would seem that healthy lifestyle choices would also reduce the risk of stroke, the fifth leading cause of death in the U.S. Researchers used data from the Women's Health Study to address this idea. The cohort included 37,636 women at least 45 years of age in 1993 when the study started; these women were followed for an average of 10 years. The healthiest behaviors were defined as: (1) never smoking; (2) alcohol consumption between four and 10.5 drinks per week; (3) physical exercise more than four times per week; (4) having a body mass index less than 22; and (5) consuming a diet high in cereal fiber, folate, and omega-3 fatty acids, with a high ratio of polyunsaturated to saturated fat, low in trans fats, and low in glycemic load. Each healthy choice was evaluated on a four-point scale. Therefore, a participant had a total score for the five healthy lifestyle choices between 0 (uniformly poor healthy choices) and 20 (uniformly excellent healthy choices). **Compared to participants with 0–4 points (revealing few healthy choices), those with 17–20 points (revealing many healthy choices) had a 55 percent lower risk of total stroke (a stroke of any kind) and a 71 percent lower risk of ischemic stroke (reduced blood flow to the brain).** No significant association was found between lifestyle behaviors and hemorrhagic stroke. For the respective healthy lifestyle choices, smoking and body-mass index were most strongly associated with a risk of total stroke[20].

Nonfatal stroke is a leading cause of permanent disability and decreased *Quality of Lifespan*. Researchers at Harvard used data from the NHS and the Health Professionals Follow-Up Study to evaluate the link between healthy choices and the incidence of stroke. At baseline, the mean age of participants was 50 years for women and 54 years for men. The researchers defined health lifestyle choices as: (1) not smoking, (2) having a moderate body mass (BMI less than 25), (3) modest alcohol consumption (5–50 grams per day for men and 5–15 grams per day for women), (4) being physically active (more than 30 minutes per day of moderate-intensity exercise), and (5) eating a good diet (scoring in the top 40 percent of adherence to the Alternative Healthy Eating Index). **Women and men who made all five healthy choices had a 79 and 81 percent lower risk of stroke, respectively, compared to those who made zero healthy choices over 18 years of follow-up. The risk of stroke for women declined in a progressive manner as the number of healthy habits increased from one to five. Men exhibited a similar pattern.** It's worth remembering that both the Nurses' Health Study and the Health Professionals Follow-Up Study involved health professionals, people who presumably adopted more healthy choices than most Americans. Thus, the beneficial effects of adopting all five of these healthy choices would likely be even greater across the entire U.S. population. Unfortunately, only four percent of the participants in both studies exhibited all five healthy choices. At least there's massive potential for improvement[21].

Reduced risk of dementia

The Lancet Commission on Dementia Prevention, Intervention, and Care recently issued a report that summarized the available literature regarding the causes of dementias and the prospects for their prevention. Quantitative analyses revealed that hearing loss (nine percent), less education (seven percent), smoking (six percent), and depression (four percent) accounted for the greatest risk. **The report concluded that up to one-third of dementia cases could theoretically be prevented. Potential interventions to prevent dementias include more childhood education, regular physical exercise, maintaining social engagement, and reducing smoking, along with managing peripheral hearing loss, depression, diabetes, and obesity. These positive outcomes could arise from *Keep Moving, Eat Better, Cultivate Social Connections,* and *Keep Learning.* Thus, we** may greatly reduce our risk of dementias if we embrace multiple healthy choices[22].

Reduced risk of chronic disease

The positive benefits documented in the Caerphilly Cohort Study may astound you. This study recorded the healthy behaviors of 2,235 men aged 45–59 at baseline in Caerphilly, South Wales. Researchers examined the relationships between healthy lifestyles, chronic disease, and cognitive decline over a period of 35 years and monitored changes in the adoption of health behaviors. The five healthy lifestyle choices included: (1) regular exercise, (2) not smoking, (3) maintaining a low body weight, (4) consuming a healthy diet, and (5) low alcohol intake. **Participants who consistently made four or five of** these healthy lifestyle choices experienced a 64 percent lower risk of dementia and cognitive decline—with exercise being the strongest mitigating factor—as well as 50 percent fewer instances of diabetes, heart disease, and stroke combined, compared with people who made no healthy lifestyle choices. Healthy choices predicted far greater beneficial effects than any medical treatment or preventative procedure. Adopting multiple healthy lifestyle choices predicted large health benefits. But this study also showed that few people followed a fully healthy lifestyle. Furthermore, the study revealed that while the number of people who smoked declined since the study started, the fraction of people who led a fully healthy lifestyle did not increase[23].

Researchers used data from the European Prospective Investigation into Cancer and Nutrition-study to see if Germans who adopted healthy choices had a lower risk of chronic disease. Between 1994 and 1998, 23,157 male and female residents aged 35–65 years of age, living in Potsdam, Germany, enrolled in the study. Four healthy choices included: (1) never smoking; (2) having a body-mass index under 30 (not overweight or obese); (3) eating a high-quality diet (lots of fruits, vegetables, whole-wheat bread, modest meat consumption); and (4) engaging in 3.5 hours of physical activity per week (more than the recommended minimum of 2.5 hours per week by U.S. health authorities). After adjusting for potentially confounding factors, such as sex, education, and occupation, compared to those participants who had zero healthy choices, those who had all four healthy choices had a 78 percent lower risk of developing a chronic disease (heart attack, stroke, diabetes, cancer) over the eight–year follow-up period. With respect to diabetes, participants who made all four healthy choices had a 93 percent lower risk compared to those who had zero healthy choices. Each of the four choices independently predicted reduced risk of chronic disease. Thus, widespread adoption of these four healthy choices could confer enormous benefits on German citizens and, presumably, for citizens in other developed countries[24].

Increased cognitive function

While smoking, physical inactivity, poor diet, and high body-mass index independently foretell poor cognitive performance, their joint effects are poorly understood. Researchers used data from 972 participants aged 23–98 years in the Maine–Syracuse Longitudinal Study to shed light on this topic. Researchers measured three health markers: total cholesterol, blood pressure, and fasting blood glucose. Each healthy choice except for diet was categorized according to the American Heart Association's definitions of ideal cardiovascular health. For diet, a positive food score (indicative of lots of fruits, vegetables, and whole grains) and a negative food score (indicative of unhealthy foods such as processed meat, full-fat dairy, and/or added sugar) were calculated. A cardiovascular health score ranging from 0 to 8 was the sum of the number of cardiovascular measures at ideal levels. Participants who had higher scores (more ideal cardiovascular health measures) also had more years of

Fats and Chronic Disease

Dr. Walter Willett at Harvard University is one of the most widely published academic experts on the health effects of what people eat. In 2006, Willett summarized his views on the connections between carbohydrates, fats, and chronic diseases. He noted that, contrary to what many lay people are told, intake of dietary fat is not significantly related to the risk of cardiovascular disease. The exhortations from the U.S. government and many nutritionists to greatly reduce fat in our diets has led to greatly increased consumption of sugar and white flour. Food manufacturers partially substituted sugar for fat in their recipes to make the low-fat foods palatable. Ironically, the drop of dietary fat and the rise in dietary sugar and white flour parallel the explosion in type 2 diabetes.

While the total amount of fat may not matter with regard to cardiovascular disease, the type of fat does. Trans fats, found in partially hydrogenated vegetable oils, are associated with an increased risk of cardiovascular disease. Increased consumption of monounsaturated oils (such as those present in olive oil) predicts a reduced education, fewer depressive symptoms, and were less likely to be on medications. **With statistical adjustment for age, education, and gender, participants' cognitive performance increased in a linear manner for seven of the eight measures of cognitive ability as the number of ideal cardiovascular measures increased from zero to eight.** Most importantly, the global cognition composite score increased significantly as health levels increased from poor to ideal for smoking, body-mass index, and physical activity[26]. Adopting the healthy choices of *Keep Moving* and *Eat Better*, along with not smoking, may improve cognitive function.

Reduced risk of type 2 diabetes

Diabetes accounts for a substantial portion of the medical care burden within the U.S., not to mention the toll it takes in human suffering. Researchers used data from 84,941 female nurses who participated in the Nurses' Health Study to evaluate the extent to which modifiable lifestyle behaviors contribute to the surge of diabetes in America. Data collection began in 1976 and continued through 16 years of follow-up. Body-mass index explained more of the risk of type 2 diabetes than any other risk factor, with 61 percent of the nurses'

risk of cardiovascular and other chronic diseases.

Increased consumption of polyunsaturated oils is also linked with better health outcomes, but, again, the types of fats in those oils matter. The ratio of omega-3 to omega-6 fatty acids affects our health. Evidence indicates that the standard American diet contains too many omega-6 and too few omega-3 fatty acids. Omega-3 fatty acids are abundant in cold water fish, a common component of some Mediterranean diets. While fiber is not a particularly sexy topic, accumulating research shows that most Americans eat far too little fiber.

Overall, Willett estimates that eating a Mediterranean-type diet, along with not smoking and regular physical activity, can reduce the risk of type 2 diabetes by 90 percent, coronary heart disease by 80 percent, and stroke by 70 percent! Imagine what would happen if we were to adopt these and other healthy choices, such as *Sleep More and Better, Cultivate Social Connections,* and *Develop a Positive Mental Attitude.* Our risk of type 2 diabetes might drop to near zero[25].

diabetes cases attributable to a BMI greater than 25. Lack of exercise, current smoking, and abstinence from alcohol were all associated with a significant risk of diabetes, even after adjusting for body-mass index. **Collectively, 91 percent of the observed cases of diabetes in this study could have been prevented by weight loss, regular physical exercise, improved diet, moderate consumption of alcohol, and not smoking**[27]. Harvard nurses could almost eliminate type 2 diabetes by incorporating just two of the nine healthy choices championed in this book, namely *Keep Moving* and *Eat Better*, and by not smoking. Imagine the result if the nurses made more healthy choices!

Type 2 diabetes is not just a problem in the U.S.—it's a global problem. For example, the incidence of type 2 diabetes in Taiwan doubled from 6 percent in 2000 to 12 percent in 2014. The recommendations for adopting health lifestyle choices based on research in the U.S. and in Europe motivated a recent study in Taiwan of the association between healthy lifestyle factors and type 2 diabetes. Subjects included 5,349 community-dwelling residents aged 55 and older. Six healthy lifestyle factors included: (1) diet (based on the Dietary Approaches to Stop Hypertension diet), (2) physical activity, (3) psychosocial health, (4) normal waist circumference, (5) not smoking, and (6) no alcohol or betel nut consumption. The incidence of type 2 diabetes declined in a dose-response manner as the number of healthy lifestyle factors increased for all age groups. **Subjects who had four of the healthy lifestyle factors (moderate to strenuous physical activity, a healthy diet, healthy psychological function, and normal waist circumference) had a 37–50 percent lower risk of developing type 2 diabetes (depending on the statistical model used) over three to five years of follow-up, compared to subjects without the four healthy lifestyle factors.** One-third to one-half of new diabetes cases could be prevented over a relatively short time period in this sample of middle-aged residents of Taiwan[28].

Reduced risk of colorectal cancer

Intuitively, it seems that people who adopt more as opposed to fewer healthy lifestyle choices would experience a lower risk of various diseases. A recent study showed this is true for colorectal cancer. Researchers analyzed data from 343,478 people living in eight European countries that have adopted a Western lifestyle. The median follow-up period was 12 years. Participants were scored on five lifestyle factors: (1) overweight or obesity, (2) physical activity, (3) smoking, (4) alcohol consumption, and (5) diet quality. Researchers found that the healthy version of each lifestyle factor independently predicted a reduced risk of colorectal cancer. **Compared to participants with no or one healthy lifestyle factor, participants with two, three, four, or five healthy lifestyle factors showed reductions in colorectal cancer of 13, 21, 34, and 37 percent, respectively. Healthy weight, not smoking, and a high-quality diet contributed most to reduced risk of colorectal cancer.** The association between healthy lifestyle and colorectal cancer was stronger for men than women[29].

Maintaining mobility in old age

The Baltimore Longitudinal Study of Aging is one of the longest-running studies of aging in the US. Aging seems to reflect progressive dysfunction of basic biological systems. **Research funded under the aegis of the study shows that healthy lifestyle choices can affect our rate of aging more than simply having more birthdays. The most important choices appear to be *Eat Better, Keep Moving,* and *Cultivate Social Connections.*** The genes we inherit from our parents account for a smaller proportion of our rate of aging. Leg strength and function predict multiple health outcomes, including reduced disability, reduced medical care utilization, reduced nursing home admission, and reduced risk of premature death. Maintaining leg strength and joint capability promote mobility, which improves *Quality of Lifespan* in old age[30].

Three Key Points

1. The more healthy lifestyle choices we embrace, the greater the benefit for our lifelong health and longevity.

2. Making multiple healthy choices over the long term can eliminate or postpone many chronic conditions and increase our *Quality of Lifespan.*

3. If many of us Americans were to make multiple healthy lifestyle choices over the long term, we could substantially reduce our personal and national medical care costs.

Summary

Create a New Normal for Your Life

This book provides an easy-to-understand, comprehensive, evidence-based approach to moving along the path of lifelong vibrant health and emotional well-being. I hope that I've convinced you—if you weren't already—that making better choices can profoundly and positively change your life. I urge you to embrace the nine healthy lifestyle choices as a new normal for your life.

More Than Diet and Exercise

The research studies summarized in this book generally focus on a limited suite of healthy lifestyle choices that includes sufficient physical exercise, a good diet, moderate body weight, not smoking, and limited alcohol consumption. While these lifestyle choices are vital and largely coincide with two of the healthy lifestyle choices presented in this book—*Keep Moving* and *Eat Better*—other healthy lifestyle choices are also important yet are typically excluded from long-term research studies. For example, *Cultivate Social Connections* may be, in fact, the most important heathy choice of all, but it's seldom included in studies of multiple healthy choices. Likewise, *Sleep More and Better* is rarely evaluated. What about *Defuse Chronic Stress*? *Keep Learning*? *Develop a Positive Mental Attitude*? *Live with Purpose*? *Participate in a Spiritual Community*? Do not conclude that these healthy lifestyle choices are unimportant because they rarely appear in research studies. All of the nine healthy lifestyle choices merit your thoughtful consideration.

Healthy Choices for Healthy Aging

Most Americans don't make many healthy choices. If you were to ask 100 people whether physical exercise is beneficial, 99 would probably say it is. Yet in spite of the widespread belief that physical exercise is good for us, only 19 percent of women, 26 percent of men, and 20 percent of adolescents meet nationally recommended guidelines for physical activity, according to the 2018 Physical Activity Guidelines for Americans published by the U.S. Department of Health and Human Services[1].

The aging of the U.S. population has potentially catastrophic consequences for the American medical care system. Translating research findings about "healthy aging" into tangible, beneficial results should be a top priority for all Americans and our public health authorities. For example, research supports the importance of *Cultivate Social Connections* with respect to later-life health and well-being, including greater longevity, cognitive function, and maintenance of daily living; lower risk of depression; and reduced risk of falling. Research also shows that *Keep Moving* is one of the strongest predictors of multiple aspects of later-life health and functioning[2]. Adopting just these two healthy choices can increase our *Quality of Lifespan*.

Healthy Changes Begin in Our Mind

In her book, *Radical Remission*, psychologist Kelly Turner[3] recounts experiences of people with cancer who were not expected to live more than a year or two, sometimes less than six months. But all of them soundly beat the odds. How did that happen? Turner speculates that survivors were more interested in living than in not dying. They had a zest for living more than a fear of dying. These cancer survivors showed that the mind leads the body, not the other way around. Survivors changed the way they saw themselves and their cancer.

A sizeable proportion of all illnesses, not just cancer, appears to arise from the mind. Perhaps this is due to chronic resentment, anger, stress, bitterness, or from being too busy. Perhaps we're so weighed down with difficulties of life that we forget our reasons for living.

Changing our belief system can change the life we experience. If we believe that we're too old, too sick, too heavy, too busy to make healthy choices, these self-imposed limitations will prevail. Alternatively, if we believe that we can make healthy choices, regardless of our age and that these choices will benefit us greatly, we can rejuvenate our life.

Get In Touch with What's Important to You

I urge you to get in touch with your deepest calling in life. If you don't have a powerful reason to keep on living, you might end up just existing, missing much of the joy that life can offer. If you identify a powerful reason for living (what I call a BIG WHY) and establish relevant, compelling goals, your life force will have direction. You will be drawn to purposeful activities that will increase meaning in your life. In my view, the best thing that you can do to move along the path of vibrant health and emotional well-being is to find an emotionally laden, powerful, and compelling reason to keep living. Identify a BIG WHY that resonates for you. Connect your big BIG WHY with making healthy choices.

In my case, while recuperating from a life-threatening accident in 2013, I identified several powerful reasons to get well and elevate my life. First, I wanted to finish the Pacific Crest Trail. Second, I wanted to experience other long-distance hiking trails and cycling adventures. Third, I wanted to share what I learned from my injury with other people so they could respond resourcefully during traumatic situations. Fourth and more recently, I felt compelled to share the power of the nine healthy lifestyle choices with others so they, too, could rejuvenate their lives.

Many factors influence how long we live. Recent research in Finland suggests that our will to live belongs near the top of that list. Finnish researchers found that elderly Helsinki residents who wanted to live much longer actually did. Residents who wanted to live at least 10 more years were twice as likely to survive over a 10-year period than those who wanted to live fewer than 5 more years, regardless of age, gender, or chronic illnesses.

Think about this: Older people who wanted to live longer *actually lived longer*. What could account for this? It wasn't the participants' age or gender or chronic conditions, because the researchers statistically controlled for them. I suspect that the people who wanted to live longer were able to *Cultivate Social Connections, Develop a Positive Mental Attitude*, and embrace other healthy lifestyle choices—consciously or unconsciously—that supported a longer and better life. The beliefs and attitudes we hold can powerfully influence how long and how well we live[4].

Small Steps Lead to Big Results

Perhaps you want to take your life to a higher level. Or perhaps you want to maintain your already-wonderful life. Whatever your reason for reading this book, I hope you have found the support and direction needed to help you move along the path of vibrant health and emotional well-being.

The research studies highlighted in this book demonstrate the *possibilities* associated with making healthy lifestyle choices. You may recall that study participants who made healthy choices reduced their risk of type 2 diabetes by over 90 percent. You can, too!

I urge you to take charge of your life. Assume 100 percent responsibility for your life. You will be motivated to embrace healthy lifestyle choices because you know they can help you achieve the life you want. In the end, the most beneficial lifestyle choice for you is the one that you actually embrace and incorporate into your daily life. Pick one of the nine lifestyle choices that most resonates with you, embrace that choice, and take action today. Make that choice an integral part of your everyday life. Small steps taken consistently over time can yield big results and help you achieve the life you want.

Endnotes

Introduction

1. Halvorson, G. 2007. *Reform Health Care Now! A Prescription for Change.* Jossey-Bass, San Francisco.

2. Miller, G. 2007. Altarum Institute. Ann Arbor, Michigan.

3. U.S. Centers for Disease Control and Prevention. Preventive Health Care – What's the Problem? Accessed April 20, 2019. https://www.cdc.gov/healthcommunication/toolstemplates/entertainmented/tips/PreventiveHealth.html

4. Ogden, C, M Carroll, B Kit, and K Flegal. 2014. Prevalence of childhood and adult obesity in the United States, 2011-2012. Journal of the American Medical Association 311:806-14.

5. U.S. Census Bureau website. Accessed April 19, 2019. https://www.census.gov/library/stories/2018/10/snapshot-fast-growing-us-older-population.html

6. Fontana, L, B Kennedy, and V Longo. 2014. Prepare for human testing. Nature 511:405-7.

7. Barbieri M, and N Ouellette. 2012. The Demography of Canada and the United States from the 1980s to the 2000s - A Summary of changes and a statistical assessment. Population (English Edition) 67: 177–280.

8. Alzheimer's Association. 2018 Alzheimer's Disease Facts and Figures. https://www.alz.org/media/HomeOffice/Facts%20and%20Figures/facts-and-figures.pdf

9. Towers Watson. 2015. U.S. Employers expect rate of increase in health care costs in 2015 to remain Low but well above inflation. https://towerswatson.com/en/Press/2015/10/rate-of-increase-in-health-care-costs-in-2015

10. Hurd, M, P Martorell, A Delavande, K Mullen, and K Langa. 2013. Monetary costs of dementia in the United States. New England Journal of Medicine 368:1326-34.

11. Schroeder, S. 2007. We can do better — improving the health of the American people. New England Journal of Medicine 357:1221-8.

12. Anand, P, A Kunnumakara, C Sundaram, K Harikumar, S Tharakan, O Lai, B Sung, and B Aggarwal. 2008. Cancer is a preventable disease that requires major lifestyle changes. Pharmaceutical Research 25: 2097-2116.

13. Herskind, A, M McGue, N Holm, T Sorensen, B Harvald, and J Vaupel. 1996. The heritability of human longevity: A population-based study of 2872 Danish twin pairs born 1870-1900. Human Genetics 97:319-23.

14. Mokdad, A, J Marks, D Stroup, and J Gerberding. 2004. Actual causes of death in the United States, 2000. Journal of the American Medical Association 291:1238-45.

15. Diener, E, and M Seligman. 2004. Beyond money – toward an economy of well-being. Psychological Science in the Public Interest. 5:1-31.

16. Willett, W. 2006. The Mediterranean diet: Science and practice. Public Health Nutrition 9:105-10.

17. Fries, JF. 1996. Physical activity, the compression of morbidity, and the health of the elderly. Journal of the Royal Society of Medicine 89:64-8.

18. Vita, A, R Terry, H Hubert, and J Fries. 1998. Aging, health risks, and cumulative disability. New England Journal of Medicine 338: 1035-41.

19. Maslow, A. 1954. *Motivation and Personality.* Harper and Brothers, New York.

20. Shonkoff, J, W Boyce, and B McEwen. 2009. Neuroscience, molecular biology, and the childhood roots of health disparities: Building a new framework for health promotion and disease prevention. Journal of the American Medical Association 30:2252-9.

21. McGill, H, C McMahan, and S Gidding. 2008. Preventing heart disease in the 21st Century - implications of the pathobiological determinants of atherosclerosis in Youth (PDAY) Study. Circulation 117:1216-27.

22. Iribarren, C, S Sidney, D Bild, K Liu, J Markovitz, J Roseman, and K Matthews. 2000. Association of hostility with coronary artery calcification in young adults. Journal of the American Medical Association 283:2546-51.

23. Everman, S, J Farris, R Bay, and J Daniels. 2017. Elite distance runners: A 45-year follow-up. Medicine & Science in Sports and Exercise 50:73-8.

24. Belsky, D, A Caspic, R Houts, H Cohen, D Corcoran, A Danese, H Harrington, S Israel, M Levine, J Schaefer, K Sugden, B Williams, A Yashin, R Poulton, and T Moffitt. 2015. Quantification of biological aging in young adults. Proceedings of the National Academy of Sciences 112(30):E4104-10.

25. Pillemer, K. 2011. *30 Lessons for Living - Tried and True Advice from the Wisest Americans*. Hudson Street Press, New York.

26. Fiatarone, M, E Marks, N Ryan, C Meredith, L Lipsitz, and W Evans. 1990. High-Intensity strength training in nonagenarians - effects on skeletal muscle. Journal of the American Medical Association. 263:3029-34.

27. Knoops, K, L de Groot, D Kromhout, A Perrin, O Moreiras-Varela, A Menotti, and W van Staveren. 2004. Mediterranean diet, lifestyle factors, and 10-year mortality in elderly European men and women. The HALE Project. Journal of the American Medical Association 292:1433-39.

28. Willis, B, A Gao, D Leonard, L. DeFina, and J Berry. 2012. Midlife fitness and the development of chronic conditions in later life. Archives of Internal Medicine 172:1333-40; Willis, B, D Leonard, C Barlow, S Martin, L DeFina, and M Trivedi. 2018. Association of midlife cardiorespiratory fitness with incident depression and cardiovascular death after depression in later life. JAMA Psychiatry 75:911-17.

29. Hamman, R, J Barancik, and A Lilienfeld.1981. Patterns of mortality in the Old Order Amish. I. Background and major causes of death. American Journal of Epidemiology 114:845-61.

30. Mitchell, B, W Lee, M Tolea, K Shields, Z Ashktorab, L Magder, K Ryan, T Pollin, P McArdle, A Shuldiner, and A Schaffer. 2012. Living the good life? Mortality and hospital utilization patterns in the Old Order Amish. PLoS ONE 7(12): e51560.

31. U.S. Department of Health and Human Services. 2018. Physical Activity Guidelines for Americans, 2nd edition. Washington, DC: U.S. Department of Health and Human Services.

32. Ory, M, and M Smith. 2017. What if healthy aging is the 'new normal'? International Journal of Environmental Research and Public Health 14(11):1389.

Chapter 1 – Keep Moving

1. Carter, G, R Hepple, M Bamman, and J Zievatle. 2016. Exercise promotes healthy aging of skeletal muscle. Cell Metabolism. 23:1034-47.

2. Rowe, J, and R Kahn. 1998. *Successful Aging.* Pantheon Books, New York.

3. Marlowe. F. 2005. Hunter-gatherers and human evolution. Evolutionary Anthropology 14:54 –67.

4. Church, T, D Thomas, C Tudor-Locke, P Katzmarzyk, C Earnest, R Rodarte, C Martin, S Blair, and C Bouchard. 2011. Trends over 5 decades in U.S. occupation-related physical activity and their associations with obesity. PLoS ONE 6(5): e19657.

5. Lanningham-Foster, L, L Nysse, and J Levine. 2003. Labor saved, calories lost: energetic impact of domestic labor-saving devices. Obesity 11:1178-81.

6. Hill, J, H Wyatt, G Reed, and J Peters. 2003. Obesity and the environment: Where do we go from here? Science 299:853-55.

7. Blackwell, D, and T Clarke. 2018. State variation in meeting the 2008 federal guidelines for both aerobic and muscle-strengthening activities through leisure-time physical activity among adults aged 18–64: United States, 2015. National Health Statistics Reports, Number 112. U.S. Department of Health and Human Services, Centers for Disease Control and Prevention, Hyattsville, MD.

8. Matthews, C, K Chen, P Freedson, M Buchowski, B Beech, R Pate, and R Troiano. 2008. Amount of time spent in sedentary behaviors in the United States, 2003–2004. American Journal of Epidemiology 167:875-81

9. Katzmarzyk, P. 2010. Physical activity, sedentary behavior, and health: paradigm paralysis or paradigm shift? Diabetes 59:2717-25; Hamilton, M, D Hamilton, and T Zderic. 2007. Role of low energy expenditure and sitting in obesity, metabolic syndrome. Diabetes 56:2655-67.

10. Segar, S, J Eccles, and C Richards. 2011. Rebranding exercise: closing the

gap between values and behavior. International Journal of Behavioral Nutrition and Physical Activity 8:94

11. Cadore, E, A Casas-Herrero, F Zambom-Ferraresi, F Idoate, N Millor, M Gómez, L Rodriguez-Mañas, and M Izquierdo. 2014. Multicomponent exercises including muscle power training enhance muscle mass, power output, and functional outcomes in institutionalized frail nonagenarians. American Aging Association 36:773–85.

12. Moore, S, A Patel, C Matthews, A Berrington de Gonzalez, Y Park, H Katki, M Linet, E Weiderpass, K Visvanathan, K Helzlsouer, M Thun, S Gapstur, P Hartge, and I Lee. 2012. Leisure time physical activity of moderate to vigorous intensity and mortality: a large pooled cohort analysis. PLoS Medicine 9(11): e1001335.

13. Hakim, A, H Petrovitch, C Burchfiel, G Ross, B Rodriguez, I White, K Yano, D Curb, and R Abbott. 1998. Effects of walking on mortality among nonsmoking retired men. New England Journal of Medicine 338:94-9.

14. Demark-Wahnefried, W. 2006. Cancer survival – time to get moving? Suggesting a link between physical activity and cancer survival. Journal of Clinical Oncology 24:3517-8; Meyerhardt, J, E Giovannucci, M Holmes, A Chan, J Chan, G Colditz, and C Fuchs. 2006. Physical activity and survival after colorectal cancer diagnosis. Journal of Clinical Oncology 24:3527-34; Holmes, M, W Chen, D Feskanich, C Kroenke, and G Colditz. 2005. Physical activity and survival after breast cancer diagnosis. Journal of the American Medical Association 293:2479-86.

15. Fang, X, D Han, Q Cheng, P Zhang, C Zhao, J Min, and F Wang. 2018. Association of levels of physical activity with risk of Parkinson disease - a systematic review and meta-analysis. Journal of the American Medical Association Network Open 1(5):e182421.

16. Ahlskog, J. 2011. Does vigorous exercise have a neuroprotective effect in Parkinson disease? Neurology 77:288-94.

17. Levine, J, N Eberhardt, and M Jensen. 1999. Role of nonexercise activity thermogenesis in resistance to fat gain in humans. Science 283:212-4.

18. McCrady-Spitzer, S, and J Levine. 2012. Nonexercise activity thermogenesis: a way forward to treat the worldwide obesity epidemic. Surgery for Obesity and Related Diseases 8:501–6.

19. DiPietro, L, A Gribok, M Stevens, L Hamm, and W Rumpler. 2013. Three 15-min bouts of moderate postmeal walking significantly improves 24-h glycemic control in older people at risk for impaired glucose tolerance. Diabetes Care 36:3262-8.

20. Cotman, C, and N Berchtold. 2002. Exercise: a behavioral intervention to enhance brain health. Trends in Neuroscience 25:295-301.
21. Deslandes, A, H Moraes, C Ferreira, H Veiga, H Silveira, R Mouta, F Pompeu, E Coutinho, and J Laks. 2009. Exercise and mental health: many easons to move. Trends in Neuroscience 59:191-8.

22. Chen, W, X Zhang and W Huang. 2016. Role of physical exercise in Alzheimer's disease (Review). Biomedical Reports 4:403-7.

23. Verdelho, A, S Madureira, J Ferro, H Baezner, C Blahak, A Poggesi, M Hennerici, L Pantoni, F Fazekas, P Scheltens, G Waldemar, A Wallin, T Erkinjuntti, and D Inzitari on behalf of the LADIS Study. 2012. Physical activity prevents progression for cognitive impairment and vascular dementia results from the LADIS (Leukoaraiosis and Disability) Study. Stroke 43:3331-5.

24. Park, B, Y Tsunetsugu, T Kasetani, T Kagawa, and Y Miyazaki. 2010. The physiological effects of Shinrin-yoku (taking in the forest atmosphere or forest bathing): evidence from field experiments in 24 forests across Japan. Environmental Health and Preventive Medicine 15:18–26.

25. Niedermeier, M, J Einwanger, A Hartl, and M Kopp. 2017. Affective responses in mountain hiking – A randomized crossover trial focusing on differences between indoor and outdoor activity. PLoS ONE 12(5):e0177719.

26. Morris, E, and E Guerra. 2015. Mood and mode: does how we travel affect how we feel. Transportation 42:25–43.

27. Oaten, M, and K. Cheng. 2006. Longitudinal gains in self-regulation from regular physical exercise. British Journal of Health Psychology 11:717-33.

28. Annesi, J. 2011. Behaviorally supported exercise predicts weight loss in obese adults through improvements in mood, self-efficacy, and self-regulation, rather than by caloric expenditure. The Permanente Journal 15:23-7.

29. Ledochowski L, G Ruedl, A Taylor, and M Kopp. 2015. Acute effects of brisk walking on sugary snack cravings in overweight people, affect and responses to a manipulated stress situation and to a sugary snack cue: a crossover study. PLoS ONE 10(3):e0119278.

30. Zehnacker, C, and A Bemis-Dougherty. 2007. Effect of weighted exercises on bone mineral density in post-menopausal women: a systematic review. Journal of Geriatric Physical Therapy 30:79-88.

31. Bolam, K, J van Uffelen, and D Taaffe. 2013. The effect of physical exercise on bone density in middle-aged and older men: a systematic review. Osteoporosis International 11:2749-62.

32. Ferrucci, L. 2008. The Baltimore longitudinal study of aging (BLSA): A 50-year-long journey and plans for the future. The Journals of Gerontology. Series A, Biological Sciences and Medical Sciences 63A:1416–9.

33. Powell, K, and S Blair. 1994. The public health burdens of sedentary living habits: theoretical but realistic estimates. Medicine and Science in Sports and Exercise 26:851-6.

34. Paganini-Hill, A, C Kawas, and M Corrada. 2011. Activities and mortality in the elderly: the leisure world cohort study. Journal of Gerontology. Series A, Biological Sciences Medical Sciences 66:559-67.

35. Barry, V, M Baruth, M Beets, J Durstine, J Liu, and S Blair. 2014. Fitness vs. fatness on all-cause mortality: a meta-analysis. Progress in Cardiovascular Diseases 56:382-90.

36. Samitz, G, M Egger, and M Zwahlen. 2011. Domains of physical activity and all-cause mortality: systematic review and dose-response meta-analysis of cohort studies. International Journal of Epidemiology 40:1382-400.

37. Medina, J. 2014. *Brain Rules – 12 Principles for Surviving and Thriving at Work, Home, and School.* Second Edition, Pear Press, Seattle.

39. Bland, J. 2014. *The Disease Delusion – Conquering the Causes of Chronic Illness for a Healthier, Longer, and Happier Life.* Harper CollinsPublishers, New York.

39. Hakim, A, J Curb, H Petrovitch, B Rodriguez, K Yano, G Ross, L White, and R Abbot. 1999. Effects of walking on coronary heart disease in elderly men - The Honolulu Heart Program. Circulation 100:9-13.

40. Hooker, S, X Sui, N Colabianchi, J Vena, J Laditka, M LaMonte, and S Blair. 2008. Cardiorespiratory fitness as a predictor of fatal and nonfatal stroke in asymptomatic women and men. Stroke 39:2950-7.

41. Rothenbacher D, W Koenig, and H Brenner. 2006. Lifetime physical activity patterns and risk of coronary heart disease. Heart 92:1319-20.

42. Kruk, J. 2007. Physical activity in the prevention of the most frequent chronic diseases: an analysis of the recent evidence. Asian Pacific Journal of Cancer Prevention 8:325-38.

43. Perera, P, R Thompson, and M Wiseman. 2012. Recent evidence for color-ectal cancer prevention through healthy food, nutrition, and physical activity: implications for recommendations. Current Nutrition Reports 1:44–54.

44. Moore, S, I Lee, E Weiderpass, P Campbell, J Sampson, C Kitahara, S Keadle, H Arem, A Berrington de Gonzalez, P Hartge, H Adami, C Blair, K Borch, E Boyd, D Check, A Fournier, N Freedman, M Gunter, M Johannson, K Khaw, M Linet, N Orsini, Y Park, E Riboli, K Robien, C Schairer, H Sesso, M Spriggs, R Van Dusen, A Wolk, C Matthews, and A Patel. 2016. Association of leisure-time physical activity with risk of 26 types of cancer in 1.44 million adults. Journal of the American Medical Association Internal Medicine 176:816-25.

45. Moreau, K, R Degarmo, J Langley, C McMahon, E Howley, D Bassett, and D Thompson. 2001. Increasing daily walking lowers blood pressure in postmenopausal women. Medicine & Science in Sports & Exercise 33:1825-31.

46. Jackson, C, G Herber-Gast, and W Brown. 2014. Joint effects of physical activity and BMI on risk of hypertension in women: a longitudinal study. Journal of Obesity 2014:271532.

47. Ogden C, C Fryar, M Carroll, and K Flegal. 2004. Mean body weight, height, and body mass index, United States 1960–2002. Advances in Data Analysis and Classification 347:1-17.

48. Cocate, P, A de Oliveira, H Hermsdorff, R Alfenas, P Amorim, G Longo, M Peluzio, F Faria, and A Natali. 2013. Benefits and relationship of steps walked per day to cardiometabolic risk factor in Brazilian middle-aged men. Journal of Science and Medicine in Sport 17:283-7.

49. Unnikrishnan, R, R Pradeepa, S Joshi, and V Mohan. 2017. Type 2 Diabetes: Demystifying the Global Epidemic. Diabetes 66:1432-42.

50. Church, T, S Blair, S Cocreham, N Johannsen, W Johnson, K Kramer, C Mikus, V Myers, M Nauta, R Rodarte, L Sparks, A Thompson, and C Earnest. 2010. Effects of aerobic and resistance training on hemoglobin A1c levels in

patients with type 2 diabetes: a randomized controlled trial. Journal of the American Medical Association 304:2253-62.

51. Pedersen, B. 2009. The diseasome of physical inactivity – and the role of myokines in muscle–fat cross talk. Journal of Physiology 587:5559–68.

52. Lanza, I, D Short, K Short, S Raghavakaimal, R Basu, M Joyner, J McConnell, and K Nair. 2008. Endurance exercise as a countermeasure for aging. Diabetes 57:2933-42.

53. Barnes D, and K Yaffe. 2001. The projected effect of risk factor reduction on Alzheimer's disease prevalence. The Lancet Neurology 10:819-28.

54. Scarmeas, N, J Luchsinger, N Schupf, A Brickman, S Cosentino, M Tang, and Y Stern. 2009. Physical activity, diet, and risk of Alzheimer disease. Journal of the American Medical Association 302:627-37.

55. Alzheimer's Association. 2015. Alzheimer's Association Report - 2015 Alzheimer's disease facts and figures. Alzheimer's & Dementia: The Journal of the Alzheimer's Association 11:332–84.

56. Hurd, M, P Martorell, A Delavande, K Mullen, and K Langa. 2013. Monetary costs of dementia in the United States. New England Journal of Medicine 368:1326-34.

57. Yaffe, K, D Burns, M Nevitt, L Lui, and K Covinsky. 2001. A prospective study of physical activity and cognitive decline in elderly women. Archives of Internal Medicine 11:1703-8.

58. Dunn, A, M Trivedi, J Kampert, C Clark, and H Chambliss. 2005. Exercise treatment for depression: efficacy and dose response. American Journal of Preventative Medicine 28:1-8.

59. Rozanski, A. 2012. Exercise and medical treatment for depression. Journal of the American College of Cardiology 60:1064-6.

60. Blumenthal, J, M Babyak, K Moore, W Craighead, S Herman, P Khatri, R Waugh, M Napolitano, L Forman, M Appelbaum, P Doraiswamy, and K Krishnan. 1999. Effects of exercise training on older patients with major depression. Archives of Internal Medicine 159:2349-56; Blumenthal, J, P Smith, and B Hoffman. 2012. Opinion and evidence: is exercise a viable treatment for depression? American College of Sports Medicine's Health & Fitness Journal 16:14-21.

61. Santilli, V, A Bernetti, M Mangone, and M Paoloni. 2014. Clinical definition of sarcopenia. Clinical Cases in Mineral and Bone Metabolism. 11:177-80.

62. Melov, S, M Tarnopolsky, K Beckman, K Felkey, and A Hubbard. 2007. Resistance exercise reverses aging in human skeletal muscle. PLoS ONE 2(5): e465.

63. Fries, J. 1996. Physical activity, the compression of morbidity, and the health of the elderly. Journal of the Royal Society of Medicine 89:64-8.

64. Fries, J. 2012. The theory and practice of active aging. Current Gerontology and Geriatrics Research. Article ID 420637.

65. Pahor, M, J Guralnik, W Ambrosius, S Blair, D Bonds, T Church, M Espeland, R Fielding, T Gill, E Groessl, A King, S Kritchevsky, T Manini, M McDermott, M Miller, A Newman, W Rejeski, K Sink, and J Williamson, for the LIFE study investigators. 2014. Effect of structured physical activity on prevention of major mobility disability in older adults - The LIFE study randomized clinical trial. Journal of the American Medical Association 311:2387-96.

66. Moreira, L, M Oliveira, A Lirani-Galvão, R Marin-Mio, R Santos, and M Lazaretti-Castro. 2014. Physical exercise and osteoporosis: effects of different types of exercises on bone and physical function of postmenopausal women. Arquivos Brasileiros de Endocrinologia & Metabologia 58:514-22.

67. Feskanich, D, W Willett, and G Colditz. 2002. Walking and leisure-time activity and risk of hip fracture in postmenopausal women. Journal of the American Medical Association 288:2300-6.

68. Kujala, U, J Kaprio, P Kannus, S Sarna, and M Koskenvuo. 2000. Physical activity and osteoporotic hip fracture risk in men. Archives of Internal Medicine 160:705-8.

69. Fiatarone, M, E O'Neill, N Ryan, K Clements, G Solares, M Nelson, S Roberts, J Kehayias, L Lipsitz, and W Evans. 1994. Exercise training and nutritional supplementation for physical frailty in very elderly people. New England Journal of Medicine 330:1769-75.

70. Hirvensalo, M, T Rantanen, and E Heikkinen. 2000. Mobility difficulties and physical activity as predictors of mortality and loss of independence in the community-living older population. Journal of the American Geriatric Society 48:493-8.

71. Nieman, D, D Henson, M Austin, and W Shaw. 2011. Upper respiratory tract infection is reduced in physically fit and active adults. British Journal of Sports Medicine 45:987-92.

72. Wang, X, B Patterson, G Smith, J Kampelman, D Reeds, S Sullivan, and B Mittendorfer. 2013. A ~60-min brisk walk increases insulin-stimulated glucose disposal but has no effect on hepatic and adipose tissue insulin sensitivity in older women. Journal of Applied Physiology 114:1563-8.

73. Mather, M, L Jacobsen, and K Pollard. 2015. Aging in the United States. Population Reference Bureau 70(2):1-23.

74. Cartee, G, R Hepple, M Bamman, and J Zierath. 2016. Exercise promotes healthy aging of skeletal muscle. Cell Metabolism 23:1034-47.

75. Puterman, E, J Lin, E Blackburn, A O'Donovan, N Adler, and E Epel. 2010. The power of exercise: buffering the effect of chronic stress on telomere length. PLoS ONE 5(5):e10837.

76. McGavock, J, J Hastings, P Snell, D McGuire, E Pacini, B Levine, and J Mitchell. 2009. A forty-year follow-up of the Dallas bed rest and training study: the effect of age on the cardiovascular response to exercise in men. Journal of Gerontology, Series A: Biological Sciences and Medical Sciences 64A:293-9.

77. Healy, G, D Dunstan, J Salmon, J Shaw, P Zimmet, and N Owen. 2008. Television time and continuous metabolic risk in physically active adults. Medicine & Science in Sports & Medicine 40:639-45.

78. Dunstan, D, B Kingwell, R Larsen, G Healy, E Cerin, M Hamilton, J Shaw, D Bertovic, P Zimmet, J Salmon, and N Owen. 2012. Breaking up prolonged sitting reduces postprandial glucose and insulin responses. Diabetes Care 35:976-83.

79. Jenkins, E, Nairn, L Skelly, J Little, and M Gibala. 2019. Do Stair Climbing Exercise "Snacks" Improve Cardiorespiratory Fitness? Applied Physiology, Nutrition, and Metabolism. https://doi.org/10.1139/apnm-2018-0675

Chapter 2 – Eat Better

1. Cordain, L, S Boyd Eaton, A Sebastian, N Mann, S Lindeberg, B Watkins, J H O'Keefe, and J Brand-Miller. 2005. Origins and evolution of the Western diet: health implications for the 21st century. American Journal of Clinical Nutrition 81:341-54.

2. Carrera-Bastos, P, M Fontes-Villalba, J O'Keefe, S Lindeberg, L Cordain. 2011. The western diet and lifestyle and diseases of civilization. Research Reports in Clinical Cardiology. 2:15-35.

3. Mann, T, A Tomiyama, E Westling, A Lew, B Samuels, and J Chatman. 2007. Medicare's search for effective obesity treatments: diets are not the answer. The American Psychologist 62:220-33.

4. Tylka, T, R Annunziato, D Burgard, S Daníelsdóttir, E Shuman, C Davis, and R Calogero. 2014. The weight-inclusive versus weight-normative approach to health: evaluating the evidence for prioritizing well-being over weight loss. Journal of Obesity Article ID 983495.

5. Tribole, R and E Resch. 2012. *Intuitive Eating: A Revolutionary Program that Works*. St. Martin's Griffin, New York.

6. Satter. E. 2005. *Your Child's Weight: Helping without Harming*. Kelcy Press, Madison, WI.

7. Eneli, I, P Crum, and T Tylka. 2008. The trust model: a different feeding paradigm for managing childhood obesity. Obesity 16:2197–204.

8. Brewer, J, A Ruf, A Beccia, G Essien, L Finn, R van Lutterveld, and A Mason. 2018. Can mindfulness address maladaptive eating behaviors? Why traditional diet plans fail and how new mechanistic insights may lead to novel interventions. Frontiers in Psychology 9:1418.

9. Mason, A, K Jhaveri, M Cohn, and J Brewer. 2018. Testing a mobile mindful eating intervention targeting craving-related eating: feasibility and proof of concept. Journal of Behavioral Medicine 41:160–73.

9. Clifford, D, A Ozier, J Bundros, J Moore, A Kreiser, and M Morris. 2015. Impact of non-diet approaches on attitudes, behaviors, and health outcomes: a systematic review. Journal of Nutrition Education and Behavior 47:143-55.

10. Estruch, R. 2010. Anti-inflammatory effects of the Mediterranean diet: the experience of the PREDIMED study. Proceedings of the Nutrition Society 69:333–40.

11. Estruch, R, E Ros, J Salas-Salvadó, M Covas, D Corella, F Arós, E Gómez-Gracia, V Ruiz-Gutiérrez, V Fiol, J Lapetra, R Maria Lamuela-Raventos, L Serra-Majem, X Pintó, J Basora, M Angel Muñoz, J Sorlí, J Martínez, and M

Martínez-González. 2013. Primary prevention of cardiovascular disease with a Mediterranean diet. New England Journal of Medicine 368:1279-90.

12. Ahmad, S, M Moorthy, O Demler, F Hu, P Ridker, D Chasman, and S Mora. 2018. Assessment of risk factors and biomarkers associated with risk of cardiovascular disease among women consuming a Mediterranean diet. Journal of the American Medical Association Network Open 1(8):e185708.

13. Guasch-Ferré, M, X Liu, V Malik, Q Sun, W Willett, J Manson, K Rexrode, Y Li, F Hu, and S Bhupathiraju. 2017. Nut consumption and risk of cardiovascular disease. Journal of the American College of Cardiology 70:2519-32.

14. Mozaffarian, D, S Kumanyika, R Lemaitre, J Olson, G Burke, and D Siscovick. 2003. Cereal, fruit, and vegetable fiber intake and the risk of cardiovascular disease in elderly individuals. Journal of the American Medical Association 289:1659-66.

15. Threapleton, D, D Greenwood, C Evans, C Cleghorn, C Nykjaer, C Woodhead, J Cade, C Gale, and V Burley. 2013. Dietary fibre intake and risk of cardiovascular disease: Systematic review and meta-analysis. British Medical Journal 347:f6879.

16. Yang, Q, Z Zhang, W Gregg, W Flanders, R Merritt, and F Hu. 2014. Added sugar intake and cardiovascular diseases mortality among U.S. adults. Journal of the American Medical Association Internal Medicine. 174:516-24.

17. Post, R, G Arch, A Mainous III, D King, and K Simpson. 2012. Dietary fiber for the treatment of type 2 diabetes mellitus: a meta-analysis. Journal of the American Board of Family Medicine 25:16-2; Chandalia, M, A Garg, D Utjohann, K Bergmann, S Grundy and L Brinkley. 2000. Beneficial effects of high dietary fiber intake in patients with type 2 diabetes mellitus. New England Journal of Medicine 342:1392-8.

18. Barnard, N, J Cohen, D Jenkins, G Turner-McGrievy, L Gloede, B Jaster, K Seidl, A Green, and S Talpers. 2006. A low-fat vegan diet improves glycemic control and cardiovascular risk factors in a randomized clinical trial in individuals with type 2 diabetes. Diabetes Care 29:1777-83.

19. Weickert, M, and A Pfeiffer. 2008. Metabolic effects of dietary fiber consumption and prevention of diabetes. Journal of Nutrition 138:439-42.

20. Salas-Salvado, J, M Bullo, N Babio, M Martinez-Gonzalez, N Ibarrola-Jurado, J Basora, R Estruch, M Covas, D Corella, F Aros, V Ruiz-Gutierrez, and E Ros. 2011. Reduction in the incidence of type 2 diabetes with the

Mediterranean diet: results of the PREDIMED-Reus nutrition intervention randomized trial. Diabetes Care 34:14–19.

21. Gu, Y, J Nieves, Y Stern, J Luchsinger, and N Scarmeas. 2010. Food combination and Alzheimer disease risk - a protective diet. Archives of Neurology 67:699-706.

22. Hsing, A, A Chokkalingam, Y Gao, M Madigan, J Deng, G Gridley, and J Fraumeni Jr. 2002. Allium vegetables and risk of prostate cancer: a population-based study. Journal of the National Cancer Institute 94:1648-51.

23. Perera, P, R Thompson, and M Wiseman. 2012. Recent evidence for colorectal cancer prevention through healthy food, nutrition, and physical activity: implications for recommendations. Current Nutrition Reports 1:44–54.

24. Bowman, G, L Silbert, D Howieson, H Dodge, M Traber, B Frei, J Kaye, J Shannon, and J Quinn. 2012. Nutrient biomarker patterns, cognitive function, and MRI measures of brain aging. Neurology 78:241–9.

25. Lourida, I, M Soni, J Thompson-Coon, N Purandare, I Lang, O Ukoumunne, and D Llewellyn. 2013. Mediterranean diet, cognitive function, and dementia - a systematic review. Epidemiology 24:479-89.

26. Valls-Pedret, C, A Sala-Vila, D Pharm, M Serra-Mir, D Corella, R de la Torre, M Martinez-Gonzalez, E Martinez-Lapiscina, M Fito, A Perez-Heras, J Salas-Salvado, R Estruch, and Emilio Ros. 2015. Mediterranean diet and age-related cognitive decline - a randomized clinical trial. Journal of the American Medical Association Internal Medicine 175:1094-1103.

27. Smyth, A, M Dehghan, M O'Donnell, C Anderson, K Teo, P Gao, P Sleight, G Dagenais, J Probstfield, A Mente, S Yusuf, ONTARGET and TRANSCEND Investigators. 2015. Healthy eating and reduced risk of cognitive decline - a cohort from 40 countries. Neurology 84:2258–65.

28. Morris, M, Y Wang, L Barnes, D Bennett, B Dawson-Hughes, and S Booth. 2018. Nutrients and bioactives in green leafy vegetables and cognitive decline - a prospective study. Neurology. 90(3):e214-e222.

29. Sonnenberg, J, and E Sonnenburg. 2015. *The Good Gut - Taking Control of Your Weight, Your Mood, and Your Long-Term Health*. Penguin Press, New York.

30. Lalia, A, S Dasari, M Johnson, M Robinson, A Konopka, K Distelmaier, J Port, M Glavin, R Esponda, K Nair, and I Lanza. 2016. Predictors of whole-body

insulin sensitivity across ages and adiposity in adult humans. Journal of Clinical Endocrinology and Metabolism 101:626-34.

31. Mozumdar, A, and G Liguori. 2011. Persistent increase of prevalence of metabolic syndrome among US adults: NAHANES III to NHANES 1999-2006. Diabetes Care 34:216-9.

32. Lerman, R, D Minich, G Darland, J Lamb, B Schiltz, J Babish, J Bland, and M Tripp. 2008. Enhancement of a modified Mediterranean-style, low glycemic load diet with specific phytochemicals improves cardiometabolic risk factors in subjects with metabolic syndrome and hypercholesterolemia in a randomized trial. Nutrition & Metabolism 5:29.

33. Weiss, R, A Bremer, and R Lustig. 2013. What is metabolic syndrome, and why are children getting it? Annals of the New York Academy Of Sciences 1281:123–40.

34. Grooms, K, M Ommerborn, D Pham, L Djousse, and C Clark 2013. Dietary Fiber Intake and Cardiometabolic Risks among US Adults, NHANES 1999–2010. American Journal of Medicine 126:1059-67.

35. Taylor, R. 2013. Reversing the twin cycles of type 2 diabetes, Banting Memorial Lecture. 2012. Diabetic Medicine 30:267-75.

36. Stokes, A, and S Preston. 2017. The contribution of rising adiposity to the increasing prevalence of diabetes in the United States. Preventative Medicine 101:91–5.

37. Basu, S, P Yoffe, N Hills, and R Lustig. 2013. The relationship of sugar to population-level diabetes prevalence: an econometric analysis of repeated cross-sectional data. PLoS ONE 8(2): e57873.

38. Sevastianova, K, A Santos, A Kotronen, A Hakkarainen, J Makkonen, K Silander, M Peltonen, S Romeo, J Lundbom, N Lundbom, V Olkkonen, H Gylling, B Fielding, A Rissanen, and H Yki-Ja"rvinen. 2012. Effect of short-term carbohydrate overfeeding and long-term weight loss on liver fat in overweight humans. American Journal of Clinical Nutrition 96:727-34.

39. Cahill, L, A Pan, S Chiuve, Q Sun, W Willett, F Hu, and E Rimm. 2014. Fried-food consumption and risk of type 2 diabetes and coronary artery disease: a prospective study in 2 cohorts of U.S. women and men. American Journal of Clinical Nutrition 100:667-75.

40. Appel, L, F Sacks, V Carey, E Obarzanek, J Swain, E Miller III, P Conlin, T Erlinger, B Rosner, N Laranjo, J Charleston, P McCarron, and L Bishop. 2005. Effects of protein, monounsaturated fat, and carbohydrate intake on blood pressure and serum lipids. Journal of the American Medical Association 294:2455-64

41. Yokoyama, Y, N Barnard, S Levin, and M Watanabe. 2014. Vegetarian diets and glycemic control in diabetes: a systematic review and meta-analysis. Cardiovascular Diagnosis and Therapy 4:373-82.

42. Pase, M, J Himali, A Beiser, H Aparicio, C Satizabal, R Vasan, S Seshadri, and P Jacques. 2017. Sugar and artificially sweetened beverages and the risks of incident stroke and dementia - a prospective cohort study. Stroke 48:1139-46.

43. Malik, V, Y Li, A Pan, L De Koning, E Schernhammer, W Willett, and F Hu. 2019. Long-Term Consumption of Sugar-Sweetened and Artificially Sweetened Beverages and Risk of Mortality in US Adults. Circulation 139:2113-25.

44. Iestra, J, D. Kromhout, Y van der Schouw, D Grobbee, H Boshuizen, and W van Staveren. 2005. Effect Size Estimates of Lifestyle and Dietary Changes on All-Cause Mortality in Coronary Artery Disease Patients - A Systematic Review. Circulation 112:924-34.

45. Hu, F, and W Willett. 2002. Optimal diets for prevention of coronary heart disease. Journal of the American Medical Association 288:2569-78.

46. Bellavia, A, S Larsson, M Bottai, A Wolk, and N Orsini. 2014. Differences in survival associated with processed and with nonprocessed red meat consumption. American Journal of Clinical Nutrition 100:924-9.

47. Rohrmann, S, K Overvad, H Bueno-de-Mesquita, and 44 others. 2013. Meat consumption and mortality - results from the European Prospective Investigation into Cancer and Nutrition. BMC Medicine 11:63 http://www.biomedcentral.com/1741-7015/11/63

48. Micha, R, J Peñalvo, F Cudhea, F Imamura, C Rehm, and D Mozaffarian. 2017. Association between dietary factors and mortality from heart disease, stroke, and type 2 diabetes in the United States. Journal of the American Medical Association 317:912-24.

49. Duffey, K, and B Popkin. 2011. Energy density, portion size, and eating occasions: contributions to increased energy intake in the United States, 1977–2006. PLOS Medicine 8(6): e1001050.

50. Rodgers, A, A Woodward, B Swinburn, and W Dietz. 2018. Prevalence trends tell us what did not precipitate the U.S. obesity epidemic. Lancet Public Health 3(4):e162-3.

51. Morris, M, J Beilharz, J Maniam, A Reichelt, and R Westbrook. 2014. Why is obesity such a problem in the 21st century? The intersection of palatable food, cues and reward pathways, stress, and cognition. Neuroscience and Biobehavioral Reviews 58:36-45.

52. Lustig, R, K Mulligan, S Noworolski, V Tai, M Wen, A Erkin-Cakmak, A Gugliucci, and J Schwarz. 2015. Isocaloric fructose restriction and metabolic improvement in children with obesity and metabolic syndrome. Obesity 24:453-60.

53. Thompson, S, B Hannon, R An, and H Holscher. 2017. Effects of isolated soluble fiber supplementation on body weight, glycemia, and insulinemia in adults with overweight and obesity: a systematic review and meta-analysis of randomized controlled trials. American Journal of Clinical Nutrition 106:1514–28.

54. Cosman, F, S de Beur, M LeBoff, E Lewiecki, B Tanner, S Randall, and R Lindsay. 2014. Clinician's guide to prevention and treatment of osteoporosis. Osteoporosis International 25:2359–81.

55. Hooshmand, S, S Chai, R Saadat, M Payton, K Brummel-Smith, and B Arjmandi. 2011. Comparative effects of dried plum and dried apple on bone in postmenopausal women. British Journal of Nutrition 106:923–30.

56. Bowden, J. 2017. The 150 Healthiest Foods on Earth: The Surprising, Unbiased Truth about What You Should Eat and Why, Revised Edition. Quarto Publishing Group USA, Beverly, MA.

57. Zhang, Y, T Kensler, C Cho, G Posner, and P Talalay. 1994. Anticarcinogenic activities of sulforaphane and structurally related synthetic norbornyl isothiocyanates. Proceedings of the National Academy of Sciences 91:3147–50.

58. Weickert, M, and A Pfeiffer. 2008. Metabolic effects of dietary fiber consumption and prevention of diabetes. Journal of Nutrition 138:439-42.

59. Pontzer, H, B Wood, and D Raichlen. 2018. Hunter-gatherers as models in public health. Obesity Reviews 19:24-35.

60. G.L. Bowman, L.C. Silbert, D. Howieson, H.H. Dodge, M.G. Traber, B. Frei, J.A. Kaye, J. Shannon, and J.F. Quinn. 2012. Nutrient biomarker patterns, cognitive function, and MRI measures of brain aging. Neurology 78:241–249; Kiage, J, P Merrill, C Robinson, Y Cao, T Malik, B Hundley, P Lao, S Judd, M Cushman, V Howard, and E Kabagambe. 2013. Intake of trans fat and all-cause mortality in the Reasons for Geographical and Racial Differences in Stroke (REGARDS). American Journal of Clinical Nutrition 97:1121–28.

61. Wells, H, and J Buzby. 2008. Dietary Assessment of Major Trends in U.S. Food Consumption, 1970-2005, Economic Information Bulletin No. 33. Economic Research Service, U.S. Dept. of Agriculture.

62. Johnson, R, L Appel, M Brands, B Howard, M Lefevre, R Lustig, F Sacks, L Steffen, and J Wylie-Rosett on behalf of the American Heart Association Nutrition Committee of the Council on Nutrition, Physical Activity, and Metabolism and the Council on Epidemiology and Prevention. 2009. Dietary Sugars Intake and Cardiovascular Health A Scientific Statement from the American Heart Association. Circulation 120:1011-20.

63. Malik, V, Y Li, A Pan, L De Koning, E Schernhammer, W Willett, and F Hu. 2019. Long-Term Consumption of Sugar-Sweetened and Artificially Sweetened Beverages and Risk of Mortality in US Adults. Circulation 139:2113-25; Taubes, G. 2016. *The Case Against Sugar.* Alfred A. Knopf, New York.

64. Gadiraju, T, J Patel, M Gaziano, and L Djoussé. 2015. Fried food consumption and cardiovascular health: a review of current evidence. Nutrients 7:8424–30; Banta, J, G Segovia-Siapco, C Crocker, D Montoya and N Alhusseini. 2019. Mental health status and dietary intake among California adults: a population-based survey, International Journal of Food Sciences and Nutrition 07: DOI:10.1080/09637486.2019.1570085.

65. Whelton, P, and L Appel. 2014. Sodium and cardiovascular disease: what the data show. American Journal of Hypertension 27:1143-5.

66. Bland, J. 2014. *The Disease Delusion – Conquering the Causes of Chronic Illness for a Healthier, Longer, and Happier Life.* Harper Collins Publishers, New York.

67. Hopkins, P. 1992. Effects of dietary cholesterol on serum cholesterol: a meta-analysis and review. American Journal of Clinical Nutrition 55:1060-70.

68. Teicholz. N. 2014. *The Big Fat Surprise: Why Butter, Meat and Cheese Belong in a Healthy Diet.* Simon & Schuster, New York.

69. Djoussé, L, and J Gaziano. 2008. Egg consumption in relation to cardiovascular disease and mortality: the Physicians' Health Study. American Journal of Clinical Nutrition 87:964–9.

70. Zhong, V, L Van Horn, M Cornelis, J Wilkins, H Ning, M Carnethon, P Greenland, R. Mentz, K Tucker, L Zhao, A Norwood, D Lloyd-Jones, and N Allen. 2019. Associations of dietary cholesterol or egg consumption with incident cardiovascular disease and mortality. Journal of the American Medical Association 321:1081-1095.

71. Cordain, L, B Watkins, G Florant, M Kelher, L Rogers, and Y Li. 2002. Fatty acid analysis of wild ruminant tissues: evolutionary implications for reducing diet-related chronic disease. European Journal of Clinical Nutrition 56:181-91.

72. Daley, C, A Abbott, P Doyle, G Nader, and S Larson. 2010. A review of fatty acid profiles and antioxidant content in grass-fed and grain-fed beef. Nutrition Journal 9:10.

73. Key, T, P Appleby, G Davey, N Allen, E Spencer, and R Travis. 2003. Mortality in British vegetarians: review and preliminary results from EPIC-Oxford. American Journal of Clinical Nutrition 78:533S-8S; Key, T, P Appleby, G K Davey, N Allen, E Spencer, and R Travis. 2003. Mortality in British vegetarians: review and preliminary results from EPIC-Oxford. American Journal of Clinical Nutrition 78(suppl.):533S-8S.

74. Kappeler, R, M Eichholzer and S Rohrmann. 2013. Meat consumption and diet quality and mortality in NHANES III. European Journal of Clinical Nutrition 67:598-606.

75. Binnie, M, K Barlow, V Johnson, and C Harrison. 2014. Red meats: time for a paradigm shift in dietary advice. Meat Science 98:445–51.

76. Larsen, T, S Dalskov, M Baak, S Jebb, A Papadaki, A Pfeiffer, J Martinez, T Handjieva-Darlenska, M Kunešová, M Pihlsgård, S Stender, C Holst, W Saris, and A Astrup, for the Diet, Obesity, and Genes (Diogenes) Project. 2010. Diets with high or low protein content and glycemic index for weight-loss maintenance. New England Journal of Medicine 363:2102-13.

77. Gardner, C, J Trapanowski, L Gobbo, M Hauser, J Ioannidis, M Desai, and A King. 2018. Effect of low-fat vs low-carbohydrate diet on 12-month weight loss in overweight adults and the association with genotype pattern or insulin secretion: The DIETFITS Randomized Clinical Trial. Journal of the American Medical Association 319:667-9.

78. Buettner, D. The Blue Zones, Second Edition. 2012. *9 Lessons for Living Longer From the People Who've Lived the Longest.* National Geographic, Washington, D.C.

79. Frassetto L, M Schloetter, M Mietus-Synder, R Morris, and A Sebastian. 2009. Metabolic and physiologic improvements from consuming a paleolithic, hunter-gatherer type diet. European Journal of Clinical Nutrition 63:947-55.

80. Jakubowicz, D, M Barnea, J Wainstein, and O Froy. 2013. High caloric intake at breakfast vs. dinner differentially influences weight loss of overweight and obese women. Obesity 21:2504-12.

81. Rabinovitz, H, M Boaz, T Ganz, D Jakubowicz, Z Matas, Z Madar, and J Wainstein. 2014. Big breakfast rich in protein and fat improves glycemic control in type 2 diabetics. Obesity Journal 22:E46-54.

82. Garaulet, M, P Gómez-Abellán, J Alburquerque-Béjar, Y Lee, J Ordovas, and F Scheer. 2013. Timing of food intake predicts weight loss effectiveness. International Journal of Obesity 37:604–11.

83. Mamerow, M, J Mettler, K English, S Casperson, E Arentson-Lantz, M Sheffield-Moore, D Layman, and D Paddon-Jones. 2014. Dietary Protein Distribution Positively Influences 24-h Muscle Protein Synthesis in Healthy Adults. Journal of Nutrition 144: 876–80; Arentson-Lantz, E, S Clairmont, D Paddon-Jones, A Tremblay, and R Elango. 2015. Protein: A nutrient in focus. Applied Physiology Nutrition and Metabolism 40: 755–61.

84. Bjelakovic G, D Nikolova, L Gluud, R Simonetti, and C Gluud. 2007. Mortality in randomized trials of antioxidant supplements for primary and secondary prevention: systematic review and meta-analysis. Journal of the American Medical Association 297:842-57.

85. Gaziano, J, H Sesso, W Christen, V Bubes, J Smith, J MacFadyen, M Schvartz, J Manson, R Glynn, and J Buring. 2012. Multivitamins in the Prevention of Cancer in Men - The Physicians' Health Study II Randomized Controlled Trial. Journal of the American Medical Association 308:1871-80.

86. Manson, J, and S Bassuk. 2018. Vitamin and mineral supplements: what clinicians need to know. Journal of the American Medical Association 319:859-60.

87. Brewer, J, A Ruf, A Beccia, G Essien, L Finn, R Lutterveld, and A Mason. 2018. Can mindfulness address maladaptive eating behaviors? Why traditional

diet plans fail and how new mechanistic insights may lead to novel interventions. Frontiers in Psychology 9:1418.

88. Schnabel, L, E Guyot, B Alles, M Touvier, B Srour, S Hercberg, S Buscail, and C. Julia. 2019. Association between ultraprocessed food consumption and risk of mortality among middle-aged adults in France. JAMA Internal Medicine oi:10.1001/jamainternmed. 2018.7289

89. Kessler, D. 2009. *The End of Overeating.* Rodale, Inc., New York.

90. DiFeliceantonio, A, G Coppin, L Rigoux, S Thanarajah, A Dagher, M Tittgemeyer, and D Small. 2018. Supra-additive effects of combining fat and carbohydrate on food reward. Cell Metabolism 28:33-44.e3.

Chapter 3 – Sleep More and Better

1. Irwin, M. 2015. Why sleep is important for health: a psychoneuroimmunology perspective. Annual Review of Psychology 66:143-72.

2. Maas, J, and R Robbins. 2011. *Sleep for success: everything you must know about sleep but are too tired to ask.* Author House, Bloomington, Indiana.

3. Beitler J, K Awad, J Bakker, B Edwards, P DeYoung, I Djonlagic, D Forman, S Quan, and A Malhotra. 2014. Obstructive sleep apnea is associated with impaired exercise capacity: a cross-sectional study. Journal of Clinical Sleep Medicine 10:1199-204.

4. Bothelius, K, K Kyhle, C Espie, and J Broman. 2013. Manual-guided cognitive–behavioural therapy for insomnia delivered by ordinary primary care personnel in general medical practice: a randomized controlled effectiveness trial. Journal of Sleep Research 22:688-96.

5. Luyster F, P Strollo Jr, P Zee, and J Walsh. 2012. Sleep: a health imperative. Sleep 35:727-34.

6. Mazzotti, D, C Guindalini, W SantosMoraes, M Andersen, M Cendoroglo, L Roberto Ramos, and S Tufik. 2014. Human longevity is associated with regular sleep patterns, maintenance of slow wave sleep, and favorable lipid profile. Frontiers in Neuroscience 6:134.

7. Yin, J, X Jin, Z Shan, S Li, H Huang, P Li, X Peng, Z Peng, K Yu, W Bao, W Yang, X Chen, and L Liu. 2017. Relationship of sleep duration with all-cause mortality and cardiovascular events: A systematic review and dose-response

meta-analysis of prospective cohort studies. Journal of the American Heart Association 6(9):e005947.

8. Taira K, H Tanaka, M Arakawa, N Nagahama, M Uza, and S Shirakawa. 2002. Sleep health and lifestyle of elderly people in Ogimi, a village of longevity. Psychiatry and Clinical Neuroscience 56:243-4.

9. Xie, L, H Kang, Q Xu, M Chen, Y Liao, M Thiyagarajan, J O'Donnell, D Christensen, C Nicholson, J Iliff, T Takano, R Deane, and M Nedergaard 2013. Sleep drives metabolite clearance from the adult brain. Science 342:373-7.

10. Rasch B, and J Born. 2013. About sleep's role in memory. Physiological Reviews 93:681-766.

11. Walker, M, T Brakefield, J Seidman, A Morgan, J Hobson, and R Stickgold. 2002. Practice with sleep makes perfect: sleep-dependent motor skill learning. Neuron 35:205-11.

12. Walker, M, T Brakefield, J Seidman, A Morgan, J Hobson, and R Stickgold. 2003. Sleep and the time course of motor skill learning. Learning & Memory 10:275-84.

13. Besedovsky, L, T Lange, and J Born. 2012. Sleep and immune function. Pflugers Archiv – European Journal of Physiology 463:121–37.

14. Westermann, J, T Lange, J Textor, and J Born. 2015. System consolidation during sleep – a common principle underlying psychological and immunological memory formation. Neuroimmunology 38:585-97.

15. Ly, J, J McGrath, and J Gouin. 2015. Poor sleep as a pathophysiological pathway underlying the association between stressful experiences and the diurnal cortisol profile among children and adolescents. Psychoneuroendocrinology 57:51-60.

16. St-Onge, M, M Grandner, D Brown, M Conroy, G Jean-Louis, M Coons, and D Bhatt. 2016. Sleep duration and quality: impact on lifestyle behaviors and cardiometabolic health - a scientific statement from the American Heart Association. Circulation 134:e367-86.

17. Drew, M, C Hoch, D Buysse, T Monk, A Begley, P Houck, M Hall, D Kupfer, and C Reynolds. 2003. Healthy older adults' sleep predicts all-cause mortality at 4 to 19 years of follow-up. Psychosomatic Medicine 65:63-73.

18. Shahar, E, C Whitney, S Redline, E Lee, A Newman, F Nieto, G O'Connor, L Boland, J Schwartz, and J Samet. 2001. Sleep-disordered breathing and cardiovascular disease: cross-sectional results of the Sleep Heart Health Study. American Journal of Respiratory and Critical Care Medicine 163:19-25.

19. Xie, C, R Zhu, Y Tian, and K Wang. 2017. Association of obstructive sleep apnoea with the risk of vascular outcomes and all-cause mortality: a meta-analysis. British Medical Journal Open 7(12):e013983.

20. Kim, E, S Hershner, and V Strecher. 2015. Purpose in life and incidence of sleep disturbances. Journal of Behavioral Medicine 38:590-7.

21. Gangwisch, J, S Heymsfield, B Boden-Albala, R Buijs, F Kreier, T Pickering, A Rundle, G Zammit, and D Malaspina. 2007. Sleep duration as a risk factor for diabetes incidence in a large US sample. Sleep 30:1667-73.

22. Holliday, E, C Magee, L Kritharides, E Banks, and J Attia. 2013. Short sleep duration is associated with risk of future diabetes but not cardiovascular disease: a prospective study and meta-analysis. PLoS ONE 8(11):e82305

23. Cooper, C, E Neufeld, B Dolezal, and J Martin. 2018. Sleep deprivation and obesity in adults: a brief narrative review. British Medical Journal Open Sport & Exercise Medicine 4:e000392.

24. Spiegel, K, E Tasali, P Penev, and E Cauter. 2004. Brief communication: sleep curtailment in healthy young men is associated with decreased leptin levels, elevated ghrelin levels, and increased hunger and appetite. Annals of Internal Medicine 141:846-50.

25. Breus, M. 2006. *Good Night: The Sleep Doctor's 4-Week Program to Better Sleep and Better Health.* Dutton Publishing, Boston, Massachusetts.

26. Markwald, R, E Melanson, M Smith, J Higgins, L Perreault, R Eckel, and K Wright. 2013. Impact of insufficient sleep on total daily energy expenditure, food intake, and weight gain. Proceedings of the National Academy of Sciences 110:5695-700.

27. Spiegel, K, E Tasali, R Leproult, and E Cauter. 2009. Effects of poor and short sleep on glucose metabolism and obesity risk. Nature Reviews Endocrinology 5:253–61.

28. Shi, L, S Chen, M Ma, Y Bao, Y Han, Y Wang, J Shi, M Vitiello, and L Lu. 2018. Sleep disturbances increase the risk of dementia: A systematic review and meta-analysis. Sleep Medicine Reviews 40:4-16.

29. Meng, L, Y Zheng, and R Hui. 2013. The relationship of sleep duration and insomnia to risk of hypertension incidence: a meta-analysis of prospective cohort studies. Hypertension Research 36:985-95.

30. Gangwisch, J. 2014. A review of evidence for the link between sleep duration and hypertension. American Journal of Hypertension 27:1235-42.

31. McGonigal, K. 2012. *The Willpower Instinct.* The Penguin Group, New York.

32. Breus, M. 2007. *Beauty Sleep: Look Younger, Lose Weight, and Feel Great Through Better Sleep.* Plume Publishing, New York.

33. Gingerich, S, E Seaverson, and D Anderson. 2017. Association between sleep and productivity loss among 598,676 employees from multiple industries. American Journal of Health Promotion 32:1091-94.

34. Rosekind, M, K Gregory, M Mallis, S Brandt, B Seal, and D Lerner. 2010. The cost of poor sleep: workplace productivity loss and associated costs. Journal of Occupational and Environmental Medicine 52:91-98.

35. Lallukka, T, R Kaikkonen, T Härkänen, E Kronholm, T Partonen, O Rahkonen, and S Koskinen. 2014. Sleep and sickness absence: a nationally representative register-based follow-up study. Sleep 37:1413-25.

36. Kanerva, N, O Pietiläinen, T Lallukka, O Rahkonen, and J Lahti. 2018. Unhealthy lifestyle and sleep problems as risk factors for increased direct employers' cost of short-term sickness absence. Scandinavian Journal of Environmental Health 44:192-201.

37. Killgore, W, E Kahn-Greene, E Lipizzi, R Newman, G Kamimori, and T Balkin. 2008. Sleep deprivation reduces perceived emotional intelligence and constructive thinking skills. Sleep Medicine 9:517–26.

38. Nebes, R, D Buysse, E Halligan, P Houck, and T Monk. 2009. Self-reported sleep quality predicts poor cognitive performance in healthy older adults. Journal of Gerontology: Psychological Sciences 64:180–7.

39. Swanson, C, S Shea, K Stone, J Cauley, C Rose, S Redline, G Karsenty, and E Orwoll. 2015. Obstructive sleep apnea and metabolic bone disease: insights into the relationship between bone and sleep. Journal of Bone and Mineral Research 30:199–211.

40. Túlio de Mello, M, F Narciso, S Tufik, T Paiva, D Spence, A BaHammam, J Verster, and S Pandi-Perumal. 2013. Sleep disorders as a cause of motor vehicle collisions. International Journal of Preventive Medicine 4:246–57.

41. American Academy of Sleep Medicine. 2015. Partial sleep deprivation linked to biological aging in older adults. ScienceDaily 10 June 2015.

42. Carroll, J, M Irwin, M Levine, T Seeman, D Absher, T Assimes, and S Horvath. 2017. Epigenetic aging and immune senescence in women with insomnia symptoms: findings from the Women's Health Study. Society of Biological Psychiatry 81:136-44.

43. National Sleep Foundation. 2015. National Sleep Foundation Recommends New Sleep Times. https://www.sleepfoundation.org/press-release/national-sleep-foundation-r ecommends-new-sleep-times

44. Harvey, A, and C Farrell. 2003. The efficacy of a Pennebaker-like writing intervention for poor sleepers. Behavioral Sleep Medicine 1:115-24.

45. Arigo, D and J Smyth. 2012. The benefits of expressive writing on sleep difficulty and appearance concerns for college women. Psychology and Health 27:210-26.

46. Tanaka, H, K Taira, M Arakawa, C Urasaki, Y Yamamoto, H Okuma, E Uezu, Y Sugita, and S Shirakawa. 2002. Short naps and exercise improve sleep quality and mental health in the elderly. Psychiatry and Clinical Neuroscience 56:233-4.

47. Green, A, M Cohen-Zion, A Haim, and Y Dagan. 2017. Evening light exposure from computer screens disrupts sleep, biological rhythms and attention abilities. Chronobiology International 34:855-85.

Chapter 4 – Cultivate Social Connections

1. Vaillant, G. 2012. *Triumphs of Experience*. Harvard University Press, Cambridge, Massachusetts.

2. Buettner, D. 2012. *The Blue Zones: 9 Lessons for Living Longer From the People Who've Lived the Longest*. National Geographic, Washington, D.C.

3. Rowe, J, and R Kahn. 1998. *Successful Aging*. Pantheon Books, New York.

4. Egolf, B, J Lasker, S Wolf, and L Potvin. 1992. The Roseto effect: A 50-year comparison of mortality rates. American Journal of Public Health 82:1089-92.

5. Wolf, S and J Bruhn. 1993. *The Power of the Clan. The Influence of Human Relationships on Heart Disease.* Transaction Publishers, Rutgers University, New Brunswick, NJ.

6. House, J, K Landis, and D Umberson. 1988. Social relationships and health. Science 241:540-5

7. Holt-Lunstad, J, T Smith, and J Layton. 2010. Social relationships and mortality risk: a meta-analytic review. PLoS Medicine 7(7): e1000316.

8. Holt-Lunstad, J, and T Smith. 2016. Loneliness and social isolation as risk factors for CVD: implications for evidence-based patient care and scientific inquiry. Heart 102:987-9.

9. Brown, S, R Nesse, A Vinokur, and D Smith. 2003. Providing social support may be more beneficial than receiving it. Psychological Science 14:320-7.

10. Inoue, S, T Yorifuji, S Takao, H Doi, and I Kawachi. 2013. Social cohesion and mortality: a survival analysis of older adults in Japan. American Journal of Public Health 103:e60-6.

11. Kim, E, J Smith, and L Kubzansky. 2014. Prospective study of the association between dispositional optimism and incident heart failure. Circulation: Heart Failure 7:394-400.

12. Diener, E, and M Seligman. 2002. Very happy people. Psychological Science. 13:81-4.

13. Uchino, B. 2006. Social support and health: a review of physiological processes potentially underlying links to disease outcomes. Journal of Behavioral Medicine 29:377-87.

14. Cherry, K, J Brown, S Kim, and S Jazwinski. 2016. Social factors and healthy aging: findings from the Louisiana Healthy Aging Study (LHAS). Kinesiology Review 5:50-6

15. Croezen, S, H Susan, J Picavet, A Haveman-Nies, W Verschuren, L de Groot, and P van't Veer. 2012. Do positive or negative experiences of social support relate to current and future health? Results from the Doetinchem Cohort Study. BioMed Central Public Health 12:65

16. Yang, Y, C Boen, K Gerken, T Lid, K Schorpp, and K Mullan. 2016. Social relationships and physiological determinants of longevity across the human life span. Proceedings of the National Academy of Sciences 113:578-83.

17. Baumeister R, and M Leary. 1995. The need to belong: desire for interpersonal attachments as a fundamental human motivation. Psychological Bulletin. 117:497-529.

18. Arhant-Sudhir, K, R Arhant-Sudhir, and K Sudhir. 2011. Pet ownership and cardiovascular risk reduction: supporting evidence, conflicting data and underlying mechanisms. Clinical and Experimental Pharmacology and Physiology 38:734–8.

19. Wood, L, K Martin, H Christian, A Nathan, C Lauritsen, S Houghton, I Kawachi, and S McCune. 2015. The Pet Factor - Companion Animals as a Conduit for Getting to Know People, Friendship Formation and Social Support PLoS ONE 10(4): e0122085.

20. McConnell, A, C Brown, T Shoda, L Stayton, and C Martin. 2011. riends with benefits: on the positive consequences of pet ownership. Journal of Personality and Social Psychology 101:1239-52.

21. Mubanga, M, L Byberg, C Nowak, A Egenvall, P Magnusson, E Ingelsson and T Fall. 2017. Dog ownership and the risk of cardiovascular disease and death – a nationwide cohort study. Scientific Reports 7:15821.

22. Kim, E, and I Kawachi. 2017. Perceived neighborhood social cohesion and preventive healthcare use. American Journal of Preventive Medicine 53(2): e35-e40.

23. Michael, Y, G Colditz, E Coakley, and I Kawachi. 1999. Health behaviors, social networks, and healthy aging: cross-sectional evidence from the Nurses' Health Study. Quality of Life Research 8:711-22.

24. Murata, C, T Saito, T Tsuji, M Saito, and K Kondo. 2017. A 10-year follow-up study of social ties and functional health among the old: the AGES Project. International Journal of Environmental Research and Public Health 14:717.

25. Kouvonen, A, R De Vogli, M Stafford, M Shipley, M Marmot, T Cox, J Vahtera, A Vaananen, T Heponiemi, A Singh-Manoux, and M Kivimaki. 2011. Social support and the likelihood of maintaining and improving levels of

physical activity: the Whitehall II Study. European Journal of Public Health 27:14-8.

26. Cohen S, W Doyle, D Skoner, B Rabin, J Gwaltney Jr. 1997. Social ties and susceptibility to the common cold. Journal of the American Medical Association 277:1940-4.

27. Rosengren, A, K Orth-Gomer, H Wedel, and L Wilhelmsen. 1993. Stressful life events, social support, and mortality in men born in 1933. British Medical Journal 307:1102-5.

28. Bennett, D, J Schneider, Y Tang, S Arnold, and R Wilson. 2006. The effect of social networks on the relation between Alzheimer's disease pathology and level of cognitive function in old people: a longitudinal cohort study. Lancet Neurology 5:406-12.

29. Tedeschi, R, and L Calhoun. 2004. Posttraumatic Growth: Conceptual Foundations and Empirical Evidence. Psychological Inquiry 15:1-18.

30. Scrignaro, M, S Barni, and M Magrin. 2011. The combined contribution of social support and coping strategies in predicting post-traumatic growth: a longitudinal study on cancer patients. Psycho-oncology. 20:823-31.

31. McDonough, M, C Sabiston, and C Wrosch. 2014. Predicting changes in posttraumatic growth and subjective well-being among breast cancer survivors: the role of social support and stress. Psycho-oncology 23:114-20.

32. Hawkley, L, and J Cacioppo. 2010. Loneliness matters: a theoretical and empirical review of consequences and mechanisms. Annals of Behavioral Medicine 40:216-27.

33. Steptoe, A, A Shankar, P Demakakos, and J Wardle. 2013. Social isolation, loneliness, and all-cause mortality in older men and women. Proceedings of the National Academy of Sciences 110:5797–801.

34. Perissinotto, C, I Cenzer, and K Covinsky. 2012. Loneliness in older persons - a predictor of functional decline and death. Archives of Internal Medicine 172:178-83.

35. Luo, Y, L Hawkley, L Waite, and J Cacioppo. 2012. Loneliness, health, and mortality in old age: a national longitudinal study. Social Science & Medicine 74:907-14.

36. Holt-Lunstad, J, T Smith, M Baker, T Harris, and D Stephenson. 2015. Loneliness and social isolation as risk factors for mortality: a meta-analytic review. Perspectives on Psychological Science 10:227-37.

37. Kim, E, A Hawes, and J Smith, 2014. Perceived neighborhood social cohesion and myocardial infarction. Journal of Epidemiology and Community Health 68:1020–26.

38. Compare, A, C Zarbo, G Manzoni, G Castelnuovo, E Baldassari, A Bonardi, E Callus, and C Romagnoni. 2013. Social support, depression, and heart disease: a ten year literature review. Frontiers in Psychology 4:384.

39. Valtorta, N, M Kanaan, S Gilbody, S Ronzi, and B Hanratty. 2016. Loneliness and social isolation as risk factors for coronary heart disease and stroke: systematic review and meta-analysis of longitudinal observational studies. Heart 102:1009–16.

40. Fratiglioni, L, H Wang, K Ericsson, M Maytan, and B Winblad. 2000. Influence of social network on occurrence of dementia: a community-based longitudinal study. Lancet 355:1315-9.

41. Saczynski, S, L Pfeifer, K Masaki, E Korf, D Laurin, L White, and L Launer. 2006. The effect of social engagement on incident dementia - the honolulu-asia aging study. American Journal of Epidemiology 163:433–40.

42. Mitchinson, A, H Kim, M Geisser, J Rosenberg, D Hinshaw. 2008. Social connectedness and patient recovery after major operations. Journal of the American College of Surgeons 206:292-300.

43. Russek, L and G Schwartz. 1997. Perceptions of parental caring predict health status in midlife: a 35-year follow-up of the Harvard Mastery of Stress Study. Psychosomatic Medicine 59:144-9.

44. Hawkley, L, and J Cacioppo. 2007. Aging and loneliness - downhill quickly? Current Directions in Psychological Science 16:187-91.

45. Greysen, S, L Horwitz, K Covinsky, K Gordon, M Ohl, and A Justice. 2013. Does social isolation predict hospitalization and mortality among HIV+ and uninfected older veterans? Journal of the American Geriatric Society 61:1456-63.

46. Valtorta, N, and B Hanratty. 2012. Loneliness, isolation and the health of older adults: do we need a new research agenda? Journal of the Royal Society of Medicine 105:518-22.

47. Baumeister, R. 1991. *Meanings of Life*. Guilford Press, New York.

48. Stillman, T, R Baumeister, N Lambert, A Crescioni, C DeWall, and F Fincham. 2009. Alone and without purpose: life loses meaning following social exclusion. Journal of Experimental Social Psychology 45:686–94.

49. Pennebaker, J, and J Smyth. 2016. *Opening Up by Writing It Down: How Expressive Writing Improves Health and Eases Emotional Pain*. Guilford Press, New York.

50. Tenney, M, and T Gard. 2016. T*he Mindfulness Edge. How to Rewire You Brain for Leadership and Personal Excellence without Adding to Your Schedule*. John Wiley & Sons, New York.

51. Nichols, M. 2009. *The Lost Art of Listening*. The Guilford Press, New York.

Chapter 5 – Defuse Chronic Stress

1. Kim, J, and D Diamond. 2002. The stressed hippocampus, synaptic plasticity and lost memories. Nature Reviews Neuroscience 3:453-62.

2. McEwen, B. 2004. Protection and damage from acute and chronic stress - allostasis and allostatic overload and relevance to the pathophysiology of psychiatric disorders. Annals of the New York Academy of Sciences 1032:1-7.

3. Jacobs, G. 2001. Clinical applications of the relaxation response and mind-body interventions. Journal of Alternative and Complementary Medicine 7S: S93-S101.

4. Cohen, S, D Janicki-Deverts, and G Miller. 2007. Psychological stress and disease. Journal of the American Medical Association 298:1685-7.

5. Taylor, S. 2010. Mechanisms linking early life stress to adult health outcomes. Proceedings of the National Academy of Sciences 10:8507-12.

6. Khoury, B, M Sharma, S Rush, and C Fournier. 2015. Mindfulness-based stress reduction for healthy individuals: a meta-analysis. Journal of Psychosomatic Research 8:519-28.

7. Schneider, R, C Alexander, F Staggers, M Rainforth, J Salerno, A Hartz, S Arndt, V Barnes, and S Nidich. 2005. Long-term effects of stress reduction on mortality in persons ≥55 years of age with systemic hypertension. American Journal of Cardiology 95: 1060–4.

8. Trafton, J, W Gordon, and S Misra. 2016. *Training your brain to adopt healthful habits: meeting the five brain challenges.* Second edition. Institute for Brain Potential. Los Altos, CA.

9. Hofmann, W, R Baumeister, GR Förster, and K Vohs. D. 2012. Everyday temptations: An experience sampling study of desire, conflict, and self-control. Journal of Personality and Social Psychology 102:1318-35.

10. Shonkoff, J, W Boyce, and B McEwen. 2009. Neuroscience, molecular biology, and the childhood roots of health disparities: building a new framework for health promotion and disease prevention. Journal of the American Medical Association 30:2252-9.

11. Stahl, J, M Dossett, A LaJoie, J Denninger, D Mehta, R Goldman, G Fricchione, and H Benson. 2015. Relaxation response and resiliency training and its effect on healthcare resource utilization. PLoS ONE 10(10): e0140212

12. Li, Q, K Morimoto, A Nakadai, H Inagaki, M Katsumata, T Shimizu, Y Hirata, K Hirata, H Suzuki, Y Miyazakf, T Kagawn, Y Koyama, T Ohira, N Takayamn, A Krensky, and T Kawada. 2007. Forest bathing enhances human natural killer activity and expression of anti-cancer proteins. International Journal of Immunopathology and Pharmacology 20:3-8.

13. Fawzy, F, A Canada, and N Fawzy. 2003. Malignant melanoma – effects of a brief, structured psychiatric intervention on survival and recurrence at 10-year follow-up. Archives of General Psychiatry 60:100-3.

14. Walton, G, and G Cohen. 2011. A brief social-belonging intervention improves academic and health outcomes of minority students. Science 331:1447-51.

15. Aldwin, C, C Park, Y Jeong and R Nath. 2014. Differing pathways between religiousness, spirituality, and health: a self-regulation perspective. Psychology of Religion and Spirituality 6:9–21.

16. Seeman, T, B McEwen, J Rowe, and B Singer. 2001. Allostatic load as a marker of cumulative biological risk: MacArthur studies of successful aging. Proceedings of the National Academy of Sciences. 98:4770-5.

17. Keller, A, K Litzelman, L Wisk, T Maddox, E Cheng, P Creswell, and W Witt. 2012. Does the perception that stress affects health matter? The association with health and mortality. Health Psychology 31:677-84.

18. Steptoe, A, and M Kivimaki. 2013. Stress and cardiovascular disease: an update on current knowledge. Annual Review of Public Health 34:337-54.

19. Dusek, J, P Hibberd, B Buczynski, B Chang, K Dusek, J Johnston, A Wohlhueter, H Benson, and R Zusman. 2008. Stress management versus lifestyle modification on systolic hypertension and medication elimination: a randomized trial. Journal of Alternative and Complementary Medicine 14:129–38.

20. Rainforth, M, R Schneider, S Nidich, C Gaylord-King, J Salerno, and J Anderson. 2007. Stress reduction programs in patients with elevated blood pressure: a systematic review and meta-analysis. Current Hypertension Reports 9:520-8.

21. World Health Organization. 2012. Dementia – A public health priority. World Health Organization, Geneva, Switzerland.

22. Wilson, R, S. Arnold, J Schneider, Y Li, and D Bennett. 2007. Chronic distress, age-related neuropathology, and late-life dementia. Psychosomatic Medicine 69:47-53.

23. Kurth, F, N Cherbuin, and E Luders. 2017. Aging mindfully to minimize cognitive decline. Journal of Cognitive Enhancement 1:108-14.

24. Picard, M, R Juster and B McEwen. 2014. Mitochondrial allostatic load puts the 'gluc' back in glucocorticoids. Nature Reviews Endocrinology 10:303-10.

25. Epel, E, S Jimenez, K Brownell, L Stroud, C Stoney, and R Niaura. 2004. Are stress eaters at risk for the metabolic syndrome? Annals of the New York Academy of Science 1032:208-10.

26. Fjorback, L, M Arendt, E Ørnbøl, H Walach, E Rehfeld, A Schröder, and P Fink. 2013. Mindfulness therapy for somatization disorder and functional somatic syndromes - randomized trial with one-year follow-up. Journal of Psychosomatic Research 74:31-40.

27. Fjorback, L, M Arendt, E Ørnbøl, H Walach, E Rehfeld, A Schröder, and P Fink. 2013. Mindfulness therapy for somatization disorder and functional somatic syndromes: Analysis of economic consequences alongside a randomized trial. Journal of Psychosomatic Research 74:41-8.

28. Daubenmier, J, J Kristeller, F Hecht, N Maninger, M Kuwata, K Jhaveri, R Lustig, M Kemeny, L Karan, and E Epel. 2011. Mindfulness intervention

for stress eating to reduce cortisol and abdominal fat among overweight and obese women: an exploratory randomized controlled study. Journal of Obesity Article ID 651936, 13 pages.

29. Chandola, T, E Brunner, and M Marmot. 2006. Chronic stress at work and the metabolic syndrome: prospective study. British Medical Journal 332:521-5.

30. Fryer, B. 2005. Are You Working Too Hard? Harvard Business Review. November 2005.

31. McGonigal, K. 2012. *The Willpower Instinct.* The Penguin Group, New York.

32. Shanahan, D, R Bush, K Gaston, B Lin, J Dean, E Barber, and R Fuller. 2016. Health benefits from nature experiences depend on dose. Scientific Reports 6:28551.

33. Dweck, C. 2016. *Mindset – The New Psychology of Success.* Ballantyne Books, New York.

34. Crum, A, P Salovey, and S Achor. 2013. Rethinking stress: the role of mindsets in determining the stress response. Journal of Personality and Social Psychology 104:716-33; Crum, A, M Akinola, A Martin, and S Fath. 2017. The role of stress mindset in shaping cognitive, emotional, and physiological responses to challenging and threatening stress. Anxiety Stress Coping 30:379-95.

35. Brooks, A. 2014. Get excited: re-appraising pre-performance anxiety as excitement. Journal of Experimental Psychology 143:1144-58; Jamieson, J, M Nock, and W Mendes. 2012. Mind over matter: reappraising arousal improves cardiovascular and cognitive responses to stress. Journal of Experimental Psychology 141:417-22.

36. Benson, H, and W Proctor. 2010. *Relaxation Revolution – Enhancing Your Personal Health Through the Science and Genetics of Mind Body Healing.* Scribner, New York.

37. Poulin, M, S Brown, A Dillard, and D Smith. 2013. Giving to others and the association between stress and mortality. American Journal of Public Health 103: 1649-55.

38. Goyal, M, S Singh, E Sibinga, N Gould, A Rowland-Seymour, R Sharma, Z Berger, D Sleicher, D Maron, H Shihab, P Ranasinghe, S Linn, S Saha, E Bass,

and J Haythornthwaite. 2014. Meditation programs for psychological stress and well-being - a systematic review and meta-analysis. Internal Medicine 174:357-68.

39. Baoa, X, S Xueb, and F Kong. 2015. Dispositional mindfulness and perceived stress: the role of emotional intelligence. Personality and Individual Differences 78:48-52.

Chapter 6 – Keep Learning

1. Roche, S. 2017. Learning for life, for work, and for its own sake: the value (and values) of lifelong learning. International Review of Education 63:623–9.

2. Bavishi, A, M Slade, and B Levy. 2016. A chapter a day: Association of book reading with longevity. Social Science and Medicine 164:44-48.

3. Baker, D, M Wolf, J Feinglass, J Thompson, J Gazmararian, and J Huang. 2007. Health literacy and mortality among elderly persons. Archives of Internal Medicine 167:1503-09.

4. Tucker, A, and Y Stern. 2011. Cognitive reserve in aging. Current Alzheimer Research 8:354-60.

5. Alzheimer's Association. 2015. Alzheimer's Association report 2015: Alzheimer's disease facts and figures. Alzheimer's & Dementia 11:32–384.

6. Leshner, A, S Landis, C Stroud, and A Downey (Editors). Committee on Preventing Dementia and Cognitive Impairment; Board on Health Sciences Policy; Health and Medicine Division; National Academies of Sciences, Engineering, and Medicine. 2017. Preventing Cognitive Decline and Dementia - A Way Forward. The National Academies Press, Washington, DC.

7. Valenzuela, M and P Sachdev. 2006. Brain reserve and dementia: a ystematic review. Psychological Medicine 36:441-54.

8. Wilson, R, P Scherr, J Schneider, Y Tang, and D Bennett. 2007. Relation of cognitive activity to risk of developing Alzheimer disease. Neurology 69:1922-20.

9. Valenzuela, M. 2008. Brain reserve and the prevention of dementia. Current Opinion in Psychiatry 21:296–302.

10. Downey, A, C Stroud, S Landis, and A Leshner. 2017. Preventing Cognitive Decline and dementia - a way forward. Sciences policy, health and medicine division, National Academies of Sciences, Engineering, and Medicine. National Academies Press, Washington, D.C.

11. Seifert, C, and A Patalano. 2001. Opportunism in memory: preparing for chance encounters. Current Directions in Psychological Science 10:198-201.

12. D Fink, L. 2013. *Creating Significant Learning Opportunities.* Jossey-Bass, San Francisco, CA.

13. Rehfeld, K, P Müller, N Aye, M Schmicker, M Dordevic, J Kaufmann, A Hökelmann, N Müller. 2017. Dancing or fitness sport? The effects of two training programs on hippocampal plasticity and balance abilities in healthy seniors. Frontiers in Human Neuroscience 11:305.

14. Blackwell, L, K Trzesniewski, and C Dweck. 2007. Implicit theories of intelligence predict achievement across an adolescent transition: a longitudinal study and an intervention. Child Development 78: 246-263.

15. Dweck, C. 2016. *Mindset – The New Psychology of Success.* Ballantyne Books, New York.

16. Miu, A, and D Yeager. 2014. Preventing symptoms of depression by teaching adolescents that people can change: effects of a brief incremental theory of personality intervention at 9-month follow-up. Clinical Psychological Science 3:726–43.

17. Mahncke, H, B Connor, J Appelman, O Ahsanuddin, J Hardy, R Wood, N Joyce, T Boniske, S Atkins, and M Merzenich. 2006. Memory enhancement in healthy older adults using a brain plasticity-based training program: a randomized, controlled study. Proceedings of the National Academy of Sciences 103:12523-8.

18. Scarmeas, N, G Levy, M Tang, J Manly, and Y Stern. 2001. Influence of leisure activity on the incidence of Alzheimer's Disease. Neurology 57: 2236–2242.

19. Malinowski, P and L Shalamanova. 2017. Meditation and cognitive ageing: the role of mindfulness meditation in building cognitive reserve. Journal of Cognitive Enhancement 1:96–106.

Chapter 7 – Develop a Positive Mental Attitude

1. Hill, N. 2015. *Think and Grow Rich*. Sound Wisdom Publishing, Shippensburg, PA; Hill, N, and W Stone. 2013. *Success Through a Positive Mental Attitude*. Ishi Press, New York.

2. Roberts, A. 1993. The power of nonspecific effects in healing: implications for psychosocial and biological treatments. Clinical Psychology Review 13:375-91.

3. Crum, A, and E Langer. 2007. Mind-set matters. Psychological Science 18:65-71.

4. Kaptchuk, T, E Friedlander, J Kelley, M Sanchez, E Kokkotou, J Singer, M Kowalczykowski, F Miller, I Kirsch, and A Lem. 2010. Placebos without deception: a randomized controlled trial in irritable bowel syndrome. PLoS ONE 5(12):e55591.

5. McKay, B, R Lewthwaite, and G Wulf. 2012. Enhanced expectancies improve performance under pressure. Frontiers in Psychology 3:1-5.

6. Bandura, A. Self-efficacy. 1994. In V. S. Ramachaudran (Editor), Encyclopedia of human behavior 4:71-81. Academic Press, New York. (Reprinted in H. Friedman [Ed.], Encyclopedia of mental health. San Diego: Academic Press, 1998); Lachman, M, and K Firth. 2004. The Adaptive Value of Feeling in Control during Midlife. The John D. and Catherine T. MacArthur Foundation series on mental health and development. Studies on successful midlife development. How healthy are we?: A national study of well-being at midlife (pp. 320-349). University of Chicago Press, Chicago, IL; Lachman, M. 2006. Perceived control over aging-related declines - adaptive beliefs and behaviors. Current Directions in Psychological Science 15:282-6; Lachman, M, S Neupert, and S Agrigoroaei. 2011. The relevance of control beliefs for health and aging. In: *Handbook of the Psychology of Aging (Seventh Edition)*. Academic Press, New York. Pp. 175-190.

7. Bandura, A. Self-efficacy. 1994. In V. S. Ramachaudran (Editor), *Encyclopedia of Human Behavior* 4:71-81. Academic Press, New York. (Reprinted in H. Friedman [Editor], *Encyclopedia of Mental Health*. San Diego: Academic Press, 1998).

8. Lau-Walker, M. 2007. Importance of illness beliefs and self-efficacy for patients with coronary heart disease. Journal of Advanced Nursing 60:187-98.

9. Sargent-Cox, K, K Anstey, and M Luszcz. 2014. Longitudinal change of self-perceptions of aging and mortality. Journals of Gerontology, Series B: Psychological Sciences and Social Sciences 69:168–173.

10. Seligman, M, T Rashid, and A Parks. 2006. Positive psychotherapy. American Psychologist 61:774-88.

11. Rozanski, A. 2014. Optimism and other sources of psychological well-being - a new target for cardiac disease prevention. Circulation: Heart Failure 7:385-7.

12. Emmons, R. 2008. *Thanks!: How Practicing Gratitude Can Make you Happier.* Mariner Publishing, Wilmington, MA.

13. Luskin, F. 2002. *Forgive for Good: A Proven Prescription for Health and Happiness.* Harper Collins, New York.

14. Lyubomirsky, S, K Sheldon, and D Schkade. 2005. Pursuing happiness: the architecture of sustainable change. Review of General Psychology 9:111-31.

15. Danner, D, D Snowdon, and W Friesen. 2001. Positive emotions in early life and longevity: findings from the nun study. Journal of Personality and Social Psychology 80:804-13.

16. Lyubomirsky, S, L King, and E Diener. 2005. The Benefits of Frequent Positive Affect: Does Happiness Lead to Success? Psychological Bulletin 131:803–55.

17. Levy, B, M Slade, S Kunkel, and S Kasl. 2002. Longevity increased by positive self-perceptions of aging. Journal of Personality and Social Psychology 83:261-70.

18. Keyes, C, and E Simoes. 2012. To flourish or not: positive mental health and all-cause mortality. American Journal of Public Health 102:2164-72.

19. Giltay, E, J Geleijnse, F Zitman, T Hoekstra, and E Schouten. 2004. Dispositional optimism and all-cause and cardiovascular mortality in a prospective cohort of elderly Dutch men and women. Archives of General Psychiatry 61:1126-35.

20. Kim, E, J Smith, and L Kubzansky. 2014. Prospective study of the association between dispositional optimism and incident heart failure. Circulation: Heart Failure 7:394-400.

21. Gump, B, K Matthews, L Eberly, and Y Chang for the MRFIT Research Group. 2004. Depressive Symptoms and mortality in men results from the multiple risk factor intervention trial. Stroke 36:98-102.

22. Kim, E, K Hagan, F Grodstein, D DeMeo, I De Vivo, and L Kubzansky. 2016. Optimism and cause-specific mortality: a prospective cohort study. American Journal of Epidemiology 185:21-29.

23. Chida, Y, and A Steptoe. 2008. Positive psychological well-being and mortality: a quantitative review of prospective observational studies. Psychosomatic Medicine 70:741-56.

24. Davidson, K, E Mostofsky, and W Whang. 2010. Don't worry, be happy: positive affect and reduced 10-year incident coronary heart disease: The Canadian Nova Scotia Health Survey. European Heart Journal 31:1065–70.

25. Boehm, J, and L Kubzansky. 2012. The heart's content: the association between positive psychological well-being and cardiovascular health. Psychological Bulletin 138:655-91.

26. Iribarren, C, S Sidney, D Bild, K Liu, J Markovitz, J Roseman, and K Matthews. 2000. Association of hostility with coronary artery calcification in young adults. Journal of the American Medical Association 283:2546-51.

27. Affleck, G, H Tennen, S Croog, and S Levine. 1987. Causal attribution, perceived benefits, and morbidity after a heart attack: An 8-year study. Journal of Consulting and Clinical Psychology 55:29-35.

28. Sun, J, E Kim, and J Smith. 2016. Positive self-perceptions of aging and lower rate of overnight hospitalization in the U.S. population over age 50. Psychosomatic Medicine 79:81-90.

29. Huffman, J, E Beale, C Celano, S Beach, A Belcher, S Moore, L Suarez, S Motiwala, P Gandhi, H Gaggin, and J Januzzi. 2016. Effects of optimism and gratitude on physical activity, biomarkers, and readmissions after an acute coronary syndrome - the gratitude research in acute coronary events study. Circulation: Cardiovascular Quality and Outcomes 9:55-63.

30. Sarinopoulos, S. 2000. Forgiveness and physical health - a doctoral dissertation summary. The World of Forgiveness 3:16-8.

31. Peterson, C, N Park, and E Kim. 2012. Can optimism decrease the risk of illness and disease among the elderly? Aging Health 8:5–8

32. Avvenuti, G, I Baiardini, and A Giardini. 2016. Optimism's explicative role for chronic diseases. Frontiers in Psychology 7:295.

33. Chopik, W, E Kim, and J Smith. 2015. Changes in optimism are associated with changes in health over time among older adults. Social Psychology and Personality Science 6:814-22.

34. Weinman, J, K Petrie, N Sharpe, and S Walker. 2000. Causal attributions in patients and spouses following first-time myocardial infarction and subsequent lifestyle changes. British Journal of Health Psychology 5:263-73.

35. Lachman, M and S Agragoroaei. 2010. Promoting functional health in midlife and old age: long-term protective effects of control beliefs, social s upport, and physical exercise. PLoS ONE 5(10):e13297.

36. Friedman, H, and l Martin. 2011. *The Longevity Project: Surprising Discoveries for Health and Long Life from the Landmark Eight-Decade Study.* Hudson Street Press, New York.

37. Levy, B and L Meyers. 2004. Preventive health behaviors influenced by self-perceptions of aging. Preventive Medicine 39:625-29.

38. Emmons, R, and M McCullough. 2003. Counting blessings versus burdens: an experimental investigation of gratitude and subjective well-being in daily life. Journal of Personality and Social Psychology 84:377–89.

39. Fuschia, S, and A Wood. 2017. Gratitude uniquely predicts lower depression in chronic illness populations: a longitudinal study of inflammatory bowel disease and arthritis. Health Psychology 36:122-32.

40. Ferrante, J, E Shaw, and J Scott. 2011. Factors influencing men's decisions regarding prostate cancer screening: a qualitative study. Journal of Community Health 36:839-44.

41. Stewart, T, J Chipperfield, R Perry, and J Hamm. 2016. Attributing heart attack and stroke to "Old Age": implications for subsequent health outcomes among older adults. Journal of Health Psychology 21:40-9.

42. Sargent-Cox, K, K Anstey, and M Luszcz. 2012. Change in health and self-perceptions of aging over 16 years: the role of psychological resources. Health Psychology 31:423-32; Wurm, S, C Tesch-Romer, and M Tomasik. 2007. Longitudinal findings on age-related cognitions, control beliefs, and health in later life. Journal of Gerontology 62B:156-64.

43. Gawronski, K, E Kim, K Langa, and L Kubzansky. 2016. Dispositional optimism and incidence of cognitive impairment in older adults. Psychosomatic Medicine 78:819-28.

44. Levy, B, M Slade, T Murphy, and T Gill. 2012. Association between positive age stereotypes and recovery from disability in older persons. Journal of the American Medical Association 308:1972-3.

45. James, P, E Kim, L Kubzansky, E Zevon, C Trudel-Fitzgerald, and F Grodstein. 2019. Optimism and healthy aging in women. American Journal of Preventive Medicine 56:116–24.

46. Kaplan, G, and T Camacho. 1983. Perceived health and mortality: a nine-year follow-up of the Human Population Laboratory. American Journal of Epidemiology 117:292-304.

47. Shirai, K, H Iso, T Ohira, A Ikeda, H Noda, K Honjo, M Inoue, and S Tsugane for the Japan Public Health Center–Based Study Group. 2009. Perceived level of life enjoyment and risks of cardiovascular disease incidence and mortality - the Japan Public Health Center–Based Study. Circulation 120:956-63.

48. Stewart, T, J Chipperfield, R Perrya, and B Weiner. 2012. Attributing illness to 'old age:' consequences of a self-directed stereotype for health and mortality. Psychology and Health 27:881–97.

49. Levy, B, J Hausdorff, R Hencke, and J Wei. 2000. Reducing cardiovascular stress with positive self-stereotypes of aging. Journal of Gerontology: Psychological Sciences 55B:205–13; Levy, B. 2009. Stereotype embodiment: a psychosocial approach to aging. Current Directions in Psychological Science 18: 332-6; Smith. J. Not dated. *Self-fulfilling prophecy – how perceptions of aging affect our later years.* Mather Life Ways, Evanston, IL.

50. Levy, B, A Zonderman, M Slade, and L Ferrucci. 2009. Age stereotypes held earlier in life predict cardiovascular events in later life. Psychological Science 20:296-8.

51. Yan, L, K Liu, K Matthews, M Daviglus, T Ferguson, and C Kiefe. 2003. Psychosocial factors and risk of hypertension – the Coronary Artery Risk Development in Young Adults (CARDIA) Study. Journal of the American Medical Association 290:2138-48.

52. Roy, B, A Diez-Roux, T Seeman, N Ranjit, S Shea, and M Cushman. 2010. Association of optimism and pessimism with inflammation and hemostasis in the Multi-Ethnic Study of Atherosclerosis (MESA). Psychosomatic Medicine 72:134-40.

53. Theresa-Freeman, A, Z Santini, S Tyrovolas, C Rummel-Kluge, J Haro, and A Koyanagi. 2016. Negative perceptions of ageing predict the onset and persistence of depression and anxiety: Findings from a prospective analysis of the Irish Longitudinal Study on Ageing (TILDA). Journal of Affective Disorders 199:132–138.

54. Robertson, D, G Savva, B King-Kallimanis, and R Kenny. 2015. Negative perceptions of aging and decline in walking speed: a self-fulfilling prophecy. PLoS ONE 10(4): e0123260.

55. Levy, B, C Pilver, P Chung, and M Slade. 2014. Subliminal strengthening: improving older individuals' physical function over time with an implicit-age-stereotype intervention. Psychological Science 25:2127-35.

56. Sheldon, K, and S Lyubomirsky. 2006. How to increase and sustain positive emotion: the effects of expressing gratitude and visualizing best possible selves. The Journal of Positive Psychology 1:73–82.

57. Meevissen, Y, M Peters, and H Alberts. 2011. Become more optimistic by imagining a best possible self: effects of a two-week intervention. Journal of Behavioral, Therapeutic & Experimental Psychiatry 42:371-8.

58. Seligman, M, T Steen, N Park, and C Peterson. 2005. Positive psychology progress - empirical validation of interventions. American Psychologist 60:410–21; Peterson, C, N Park, and M Seligman. 2004. Strengths of character and well-being. Journal of Social and Clinical Psychology 23:603-19.

59. Pennebaker, J, and J Smythe. 2016. *Opening Up by Writing It Down, Third Edition: How Expressive Writing Improves Health and Eases Emotional Pain.* Guilford Press, New York.

60. Niedermeier, M, J Einwanger, A Hartl, and M Kopp. 2017. Affective responses in mountain hiking – A randomized crossover trial focusing on differences between indoor and outdoor activity. PLoS ONE 12(5): e0177719.

61. Tenney, M, and T Gard. 2016. *The Mindfulness Edge. How to Rewire You Brain for Leadership and Personal Excellence without Adding to Your Schedule.* John Wiley & Sons, New York.

62. Christakis, N and J Fowler, 2007. The spread of obesity in a large social network over 32 years. New England Journal of Medicine 357:370-7.

Chapter 8 – Live with Purpose

1. Leider, R. 2010. The Power of Purpose: Find Meaning, Live Longer, Better. Berrett-Koehler Publishers, Oakland, CA.

2. Seligman, M. 2011. Flourish: A Visionary New Understanding of Happiness and Well-being. Free Press, New York.

3. Amabile, T, and S Kramer. Inner work life: Understanding the subtext of business performance. Harvard Business Review May 2007.

4. Sharkey, L, and M Barrett. 2017. The Future-proof Workplace: Six Strategies to Accelerate Talent Development, Reshape Your Culture, and Succeed with Purpose. John Wiley & Sons, New York.   Hoboken, NJ.

5. Nuer, L. 2000. Learning as leadership: a methodology for organizational change through personal mastery. Performance Improvement 38:9-13.

6. Pillemer, K. 2012. 30 Lessons for Living: Tried and True Advice from the Wisest Americans. Avery, New York.

7. Roepke, A, E Jayawickreme, and O Riffle. 2014. Meaning and health: a systematic review. Applied Research Quality Life 9:1055.

8. Hill, P, and N Turiano. 2014. Purpose in life as a predictor of mortality across adulthood. Psychological Science 25:1482-6.

9. Langer, E, and J Rodin. 1976. The effects of choice and enhanced personal responsibility for the aged: a field experiment in an institutional setting. Journal of Personality and Social Psychology 34:191-8; Rodin, J, and E Langer. 1977. Long-term effects of a control-relevant intervention with the institutionalized aged. Journal of Personality and Social Psychology 35:897-902.

10. Okun, M, E Yeung, and S Brown. 2013. Volunteering by older adults and risk of mortality: a meta-analysis. Psychology and Aging 28:564–77.

11. Glass, T, C Mendes de Leon, R Marottoli, and L Berkman. 1999. Population based study of social and productive activities as predictors of survival among elderly Americans. British Medical Journal 319:478-83.

12. Krause, N. 2009. Meaning in life and mortality. Journal of Gerontology: Social Sciences, 64B:517–27.

13. Steptoe, A, A Deaton, and A Stone. 2015. Subjective wellbeing, health, and ageing. Lancet 385:640–8.

14. Zilioli, S, R Slatcher, A Ong, and T Gruenewald. 2015. Purpose in life predicts allostatic load ten years later. Journal of Psychosomatic Research 79:451–57.

15. Yang, Q, X Tong, L Schieb, A Vaughan, C Gillespie, J Wiltz, S King, E Odom, R Merritt, Y Hong, and M George. 2017. Vital Signs: recent trends in stroke death rates - United States, 2000–2015. Morbidity and Mortality Weekly Report 2017 66:933–9.

16. Kim, E, J Sun, N Park, and C Peterson. 2013. Purpose in life and reduced incidence of stroke in older adults: "The Health and Retirement Study". Journal of Psychosomatic Research 74:427-32.

17. Cohen, R, C Bavishi, and A Rozanski. 2016. Purpose in life and its relationship to all-cause mortality and cardiovascular events: a meta-analysis. Psychosomatic Medicine 78:122-33.

18. Schreier, H, K Schonert-Reichl, and E Chen. 2013. Effect of volunteering on risk factors for cardiovascular disease in adolescents - a randomized controlled trial. Journal of the American Medical Association Pediatrics 167:327-32.

19. Steger, M, A Fitch-Martin, J Donnelly, and K Rickard. 2015. Meaning in life and health: proactive health orientation links meaning in life to health variables among american undergraduates. Journal of Happiness Studies 16:583–97.

20. Yeung, J, Z Zhang, and T Kim. 2018. Volunteering and health benefits in general adults: cumulative effects and forms. BioMed Central Public Health 18:8.

21. Schwartz, C, J Meisenhelder, Y Ma, and G Reed. 2003. Altruistic social interest behaviors are associated with better mental health. Psychosomatic Medicine 65:778-85.

22. Boyle, P, A Buchman, and D Bennett. 2010. Purpose in life is associated with a reduced risk of incident disability among community-dwelling older persons. American Journal of Geriatric Psychiatry 18:1093–1002.

23. Boyle, P, A Buchman, L Barnes, and D Bennett. 2010. Effect of a purpose in life on risk of incident Alzheimer disease and mild cognitive impairment in community-dwelling older persons. Archives of General Psychiatry 67:304–10; Boyle, P, A Buchman, R Wilson, L Yu, J Schneider, and D Bennett. 2012. Effect of purpose in life on the relation between Alzheimer disease pathologic changes on cognitive function in advanced age. Archives of General Psychiatry 69:499-506.

24. Morrow-Howell, N, J Hinterlong, P Rozario, and F Tang. 2003. Effects of volunteering on the well-being of older adults. Journal of Gerontology: Social Sciences 58B:S137–45.

25. Schwingel, A, M Niti, C Tang, and T Ng. 2009. Continued work employment and volunteerism and mental well-being of older adults: Singapore longitudinal ageing studies. Age and Ageing 38: 531–7.

26. Steger, M, S Oishi, and T Kashdan. 2009. Meaning in life across the life span: levels and correlates of meaning in life from emerging adulthood to older adulthood. The Journal of Positive Psychology 4:43–52.

27. Kashihara, D, and K Carper. 2012. National health care expenses in the U.S. civilian noninstitutionalized population, 2009. Agency for Healthcare Research and Quality, No. 355.

28. Kim, E, N Park, and C Peterson. 2014. Dispositional optimism protects older adults from stroke: The Health and Retirement Study. Stroke 42:2855-9.

29. Kim, E, and S Konrath. 2016. Volunteering is prospectively associated with health care use among older adults. Social Science & Medicine 149:122-9.

30. Kim, E, I Kawachi, Y Chen, and L Kubzansky. 2017. Association between purpose in life and objective measures of physical function in older adults. JAMA Psychiatry 74:1039-45.

31. Mogilner, C, Z Chance, and M Norton. 2012. Giving time gives you time. Psychological Science 23:1233-8.

32. Piko, B, L Brassai, and M Steger. 2015. A reason to stay healthy: the role of meaning in life in relation to physical activity and healthy eating among adolescents. Journal of Health Psychology 20:473-82.

33. Pillemer, K, T Fuller-Rowell, M Reid, and N Wells. 2010. Environmental volunteering and health outcomes over a 20-year period. The Gerontologist 50:594-602.

34. Kim, E, S Hershner, and V Strecher. 2015. Purpose in life and incidence of sleep disturbances. Journal of Behavioral Medicine 38:590-7.

35. Powell, T, R Gilson, and C Collin. 2012. TBI 13 years on: factors associated with post-traumatic growth. Disability and Rehabilitation 34:1461-7.

36. Middleton, H. 2016. Flourishing and posttraumatic growth. An empirical take on ancient wisdoms. Health Care Analysis 24:133–47.

37. Tedeschi, R, and L Calhoun. 1995. *Trauma and Transformation: Growing in the Aftermath of Suffering.* Sage Publications, Thousand Oaks, CA; Peterson, C, N Park, N Pole, W D'Andrea, and M Seligman. 2008. Strengths of character and posttraumatic growth. Journal of Traumatic Stress 21:214–17.

38. Sone, T, N Nakaya, K Ohmori, T Shimazu, M Higashiguchi, M Kakiz, N Kikuchi, S Kuriyama, and I Tsuji. 2008. Sense of life worth living (*ikigai*) and mortality in Japan: Ohsaki Study. Psychosomatic Medicine 70:709-15.

39. Britton, A and M Shipley. 2010. Bored to death? International Journal of Epidemiology 39:370-1.

40. Tomioka, K, N Kurumatani, and H Hosoi. 2016. Relationship of having hobbies and a purpose in life with mortality, activities of daily living, and instrumental activities of daily living among community-dwelling elderly adults. Journal of Epidemiology 26:361-70.

41. Shin, J, and M Steger. Promoting Meaning and Purpose in Life. 2014. Pp. 90-123 in Acacia C. Parks and Stephen M. Schueller (Editors) *The Wiley Blackwell handbook of Positive Psychological Interventions, First Edition.* John Wiley & Sons, New York.

42. Schmuck, P, T Kasser, and R Ryan. 2000. Intrinsic and extrinsic goals: their structure and relationship to well-being in German and U.S. college students. Social Indicators Research 50:225-41; Weinstein, N, A Przybylski, and R Ryan. 2009. Can nature make us more caring? Effects of immersion in nature on

intrinsic aspirations and generosity. Personality and Social Psychology Bulletin 35:1315-29.

43. Dunn, L, M Norton, and L Aknin. 2008. Spending money on other promotes happiness. Science 319:1687-8.

Chapter 9 – Participate in a Spiritual Community

1. Aldwin, C, C Park, Y Jeong, and R Nath. 2014. Differing pathways between religiousness, spirituality, and health: a self-regulation perspective. Psychology of Religion and Spirituality 6:9–21.

2. Koenig, H. 2012. Religion, spirituality, and health: the research and clinical implications. International Scholarly Research Network Psychiatry. Article ID 278730

3. Gallup Organization. 2017 Update on Americans and religion. https://news.gallup.com/poll/224642/2017-update-americans-religion.aspx

4. Strawbridge, W, R Cohen, S Shema, and G Kaplan. 1997. Frequent attendance at religious services and mortality over 28 years. American Journal of Public Health 87:957-61.

5. Koenig, H, J Hays, D Larson, L George, H Cohen, M McCullough, K Meador, and D Blazer. 1999. Does religious attendance prolong survival? A six-year follow-up study of 3,968 older adults. Journal of Gerontology: Medical Sciences 54A:M370-6.

6. McCullough, M, W Hoyt, D Larson, H Koenig, and C Thoresen. 2000. Religious involvement and mortality: a meta-analytic review. Health Psychology 19:211-22.

7. Li, S, M Stampfer, D Williams, and T VanderWeele. 2016. Association of religious service attendance with mortality among women. Journal of the American Medical Association Internal Medicine 176:777-85.

8. Kim, E, and T VanderWeele. 2019. Mediators of the association between religious service attendance and mortality. American Journal of Epidemiology 188:96-101.

9. VanderWeele, T, J Yu, Y Cozier, L Wise, M Argentieri, L Rosenberg, J Palmer, and A Shields. 2017. Attendance at religious services, prayer, religious coping,

and religious/spiritual identity as predictors of all-cause mortality in the black women's health study. American Journal of Epidemiology 185:515-22.

10. Koenig, H. 2009. Research on religion, spirituality, and mental health: a review. Canadian Journal of Psychiatry 54:283-91.

11. Park, C. 2013. The meaning making model: a framework for understanding meaning, spirituality, and stress-related growth in health psychology. The European Health Psychologist 15:40-7.

12. Gillum, R, and D Ingram. 2006. Frequency of attendance at religious services, hypertension, and blood pressure: the Third National Health and Nutrition Examination Survey. Psychosomatic Medicine 68:382–5.

13. Mochon, D, M Norton, and D Ariely. 2008. Getting off the hedonic treadmill, one step at a time: the impact of regular religious practice and exercise on well-being. Journal of Economic Psychology 29:632–42.

14. Koenig, H. 2015. Religion, spirituality, and health: a review and update. Advances in Mind Body Medicine 29:19-26.

15. VanderWeele, T, S Li, A Tsai, and I Kawachi. 2016. Association Between Religious Service Attendance and Lower Suicide Rates Among US Women. Journal of the American Medical Association Psychiatry 73:845-51.

16. Strawbridge, W, S Shema, R Cohen, and G Kaplan. 2001. Religious attendance increases survival by improving and maintaining good health behaviors, mental health, and social relationships. Annals of Behavioral Medicine. 23:68-74.

17. Ironson, G, R Stuetzle, and M Fletcher. 2006. An increase in religiousness/spirituality occurs after HIV diagnosis and predicts slower disease progression over 4 years in people with HIV. Journal of General Internal Medicine 21:S62-8.

18. Bruce, M, D Martins, K Duru, B Beech, M Sims, N Harawa, R Vargas, D Kermah, S Nicholas, A Brown, and K Norris. 2017. Church attendance, allostatic load and mortality in middle aged adults. PLoS ONE 12(5): e0177618.

19. Gillum, R. 2006. Frequency of attendance at religious services and leisure-time physical activity in American women and men: the Third National Health and Nutrition Examination Survey. Annals of Behavioral Medicine 31:30–35.

20. Cornah, D. 2006. The impact of spirituality on mental health. A review of the literature. The Mental Health Foundation, London.

21. Ellison, C, A Burdette, and T Hill. 2009. Blessed assurance: religion, anxiety, and tranquility among US adults. Social Science Research 38:656-67.

22. Reeves, R, A Beazley, and C Adams. 2011. Religion and Spirituality: Can It Adversely Affect Mental Health Treatment? Journal of Psychosocial Nursing and Mental Health Services 49:6-7.

23. VanderWeele, T, J Yu, Y Cozier, L Wise, M Argentieri, L Rosenberg, J Palmer, and A Shields. 2017. Attendance at Religious Services, Prayer, Religious Coping, and Religious/Spiritual Identity as Predictors of All-Cause Mortality in the Black Women's Health Study. American Journal of Epidemiology 185:515-22.

24. VanderWeele, T, T Balboni, and H Koh. 2017. Health and spirituality. Journal of the American Medical Association 318:519-20.

Chapter 10 – Benefits of Multiple Healthy Lifestyle Choices

1. Newberg, A, and M Waldman. 2009. *How God Changes Your Brain*. Ballantyne Books, New York.

2. Housman, J, and S Dorman. 1992. The Alameda County Study: a systematic, chronological review. American Journal of Health Education 36:302-8.

3. Byrne, D, L Rolando, M Aliyu ,P McGown, L Connor, B Awalt, M Holmes, L Wang, and M Yarbrough. 2016. Modifiable healthy lifestyle behaviors: 10-year health outcomes from a health promotion program. American Journal of Preventive Medicine 51:1027–37.

4. Walsh, R. 2011. Lifestyle and mental health. American Psychologist 66:579-92.

5. Willcox, B, Q He, R Chen, K Yano, K Masaki, J Grove, T Donlon, D Willcox, and J Curb. 2006. Midlife risk factors and healthy survival in men. Journal of the American Medical Association 296:2343-50.

6. Yates, L, L Djousse, T Kurth, J Buring, and J Gaziano. 2008. Exceptional longevity in men modifiable factors associated with survival and function to age 90 Years. Archives of Internal Medicine 168:284-90.

7. Khaw, K, N Wareham, S Bingham, A Welch, R Luben, and N Day. 2008. Combined impact of health behaviours and mortality in men and women: the EPIC-Norfolk Prospective Population Study. PLoS ONE Medicine 5(1):e12.

8. Loef, M, and H Walach. 2012. Fruit, vegetables and prevention of cognitive decline or dementia: a systematic review of cohort studies. The Journal of N utrition, Health & Aging 16: 626-30.

9. Chiuve, S, T Fung, K Rexrode, D Spiegelman, J Manson, M Stampfer, and C Albert. 2011. Adherence to a low-risk, healthy lifestyle and risk of sudden cardiac death among women. Journal of the American Medical Association 306:62-69.

10. Rizzuto, D, N Orsini, C Qiu, H Wang, and L Fratiglioni. 2012. Lifestyle, social factors, and survival after age 75: population based study. British Medical Journal 345:e5568.

11. Stampfer, M, F Hu, J Manson, E Rimm, and W Willett. 2000. Primary prevention of coronary heart disease in women through diet and lifestyle. New England Journal of Medicine 343:6-22.

12. Lloyd-Jones, D, E Leip, M Larson, R D'Agostino, A Beiser, P Wilson, P Wolf, and D Levy. 2006. Prediction of lifetime risk for cardiovascular disease by risk factor burden at 50 years of age. Circulation 113:791-8.

13. Loprinzi, P, A Branscum, J Hanks, and E Smit. 2016. Healthy lifestyle characteristics and their joint association with cardiovascular disease biomarkers in U.S. adults. Mayo Clinic Proceedings 91:432-42.

14. Chiuve, S, M McCullough, F Sacks, and E Rimm. 2006. Healthy lifestyle factors in the primary prevention of coronary heart disease among men - benefits among users and nonusers of lipid-lowering and antihypertensive medications. Circulation 114:160-7.

15. Ahmed, H, M Blaha, K Nasir, S Jones, J Rivera, A Agatston, R Blankstein, N Wong, S Lakoski, M Budoff, G Burke, C Sibley, P Ouyang, and R Blumenthal. 2013. Low-risk lifestyle, coronary calcium, cardiovascular events, and mortality: results from MESA. American Journal of Epidemiology 178:12-21.

16. Ornish, D, S Brown, L Scherwitz, J Billings, W Armstrong, T Ports, S McLanahan, R Kirkeeide, R Brand, and K Gould. 1990. Can lifestyle changes reverse coronary heart disease? Lancet 336:129-33.

17. Koertge, J, G Weidner, M Elliott-Eller, L Scherwitz, T Merritt-Worden, R Marlin, L Lipsenthal, M Guarneri, R Finkel, D Saunders, P McCormac, J Scheer, R Collins, and D Ornish. 2003. Improvement in medical risk factors and quality of life in women and men with coronary artery disease in the Multicenter Lifestyle Demonstration Project. American Journal of Cardiology 91:1316 –22.

18. Silberman, A, R Banthia, I Estay, C Kemp, J Studley, D Hereras, and D Ornish. 2010. The effectiveness and efficacy of an intensive cardiac rehabilitation program in 24 sites. American Journal of Health Prevention 24:260-6.

19. Govil, S, G Weidner, T Merritt-Worden, and D Ornish. 2009. Socioeconomic status and improvements in lifestyle, coronary risk factors, and quality of life: the Multisite Cardiac Lifestyle Intervention Program. American Journal of Public Health 99:1263-70.

20. Kurth, T, S Moore, J Gaziano, C Kase, M Stampfer, K Berger, and J Buring. 2006. Healthy lifestyle and the risk of stroke in women. Archives of Internal Medicine 166:1403-9.

21. Chiuve, S, K Rexrode, D Spiegelman, G Logroscino, J Manson, and E Rimm. 2008. Primary prevention of stroke by healthy lifestyle. Circulation. 118:947-54.

22. Livingston, G, A Sommerlad, V Orgeta, S Costafreda, J Huntley, D Ames, C Ballard, S Banerjee, A Burns, J Cohen-Mansfield, C Cooper, N Fox, L Gitlin, R Howard, H Kales, E Larson, K Ritchie, K Rockwood, E Sampson, Q Samus, L Schneider, G Selbæk, L Teri, and N Mukadam. 2017. Dementia prevention, intervention, and care. Lancet 390:10113.

23. Elwood, P, J Galante, J Pickering, S Palmer, Y Ben-Shlomo, M Longley, and J Gallacher. 2013. Healthy lifestyles reduce the incidence of chronic diseases and dementia: evidence from the Caerphilly Cohort Study. PLoS ONE 8(12): 1-7.

24. Ford, E, M Bergmann, J Kröger, A Schienkiewitz, C Weikert, and H Boeing. 2009. Healthy living is the best revenge findings from the European Prospective Investigation Into Cancer and Nutrition–Potsdam Study. Archives of Internal Medicine 169:1355-62

25. Willett, W. 2006. The Mediterranean diet: science and practice. Public Health Nutrition 9:105-10.

26.Crichton, G, M Elias, A Davey, and A Alkerwi. 2014. Cardiovascular health and cognitive function: the Maine-Syracuse Longitudinal Study. PLoS ONE 9(3):e89317.

27. Hu, F, J Mason, M Stampfer, G Colditz, S Liu, C Solomon, and W Willett. 2001. Diet, lifestyle, and the risk of type 2 diabetes mellitus in women. New England Journal of Medicine 345:790-7.

28. Chen, C, K Liu, C Hsu, H Chang, H Chung, J Liu, Y Liu, T Tsai, W Liaw, I Lin, H Wu, C Juan, H Chiu, M Lee, and C Hsiung. 2017. Healthy lifestyle and normal waist circumference are associated with a lower 5-year risk of type 2 diabetes in middle-aged and elderly individuals Results from the healthy aging longitudinal study in Taiwan (HALST). Medicine 96:6(e6025)

29. Aleksandrova, K, T Pischon, M Jenab, H Bueno-de-Mesquita, V Fedirko, T Norat, and 41 others. 2014. Combined impact of healthy lifestyle factors on colorectal cancer: a large European cohort study. BioMed Central Medicine 12:168.

30. Ferrucci, L. 2008. The Baltimore Longitudinal Study of Aging (BLSA): a 50-year-long journey and plans for the future. Journal of Gerontology: Medical Sciences 63A:1416–9.

Summary

1. U.S. Department of Health and Human Services. *Physical Activity Guidelines for Americans, 2nd edition.* Washington, DC: U.S. Department of Health and Human Services; 2018.

2. Ory, M, and M Smith. 2017. What if healthy aging is the 'new normal'? International Journal of Environmental Research and Public Health 14(11): 1389.

3. Turner, K. 2014. *Radical Remission: Surviving Cancer Against All Odds.* HarperCollins Publishers, New York.

4. Karppinen, H, M Laakkonen, T Strandberg, R Tilvis, and K Pitkaka. 2012. Will-to-live and survival in a 10-year follow-up among older people. Age and Ageing 41: 789–94.

Recommended Resources

Anderson, N. 2003. *Emotional Longevity – What Really Determines How Long You Will Live.* Penguin Books, New York.

Bortz, W. 2010. *The Roadmap to 100: The Breakthrough Science of Living a Long and Healthy Life.* Palgrave Macmillan, New York.

Bowden, J. 2007. *The 150 Healthiest Foods on Earth: The Surprising, Unbiased Truth about What You Should Eat and Why.* Fair Winds Press, Beverly, MA.

Breus, M. *Beauty Sleep: Look Younger, Lose Weight, and Feel Great Through Better Sleep.* 2007. Plume Books, New York.

Buettner, D. 2012. *The Blue Zones: 9 Lessons for Living Longer from the People Who've Lived the Longest.* Second Edition. National Geographic Society, Washington, DC.

Crowley, C, and H Lodge. 2004. *Younger Next Year: Live Strong, Fit, and Sexy - Until You're 80 and Beyond.* Workman Publishing, New York.

Emmons, R. 2007. *Thanks! How the New Science of Gratitude Can Make You Happier.* Houghton Mifflin Company, New York.

Friedman, H and L Martin. 2011. *The Longevity Project – Surprising Discoveries for Health and Long Life from the Landmark Eight-decade Study.* Hudson Street Press, New York.

Luskin, F. 2003. *Forgive for Good: A Proven Prescription for Health and Happiness.* HarperColllins, San Francisco.

Lyubomirsky, S. 2010. *The How of Happiness: A Scientific Approach to Getting the Life You Want.* Penguin Press, New York.

Medina, J. 2014. *Brain Rules: 12 Principles for Surviving and Thriving at Work, Home, and School.* Updated and expanded. Pear Press, Seattle. WA.

Pennebaker, J, and J Smyth. 2016. *Opening Up by Writing It Down – How Expressive Writing Improves Health and Eases Emotional Pain.* Third Edition. The Guilford Press, New York.

Pillemer, K. 2011. *30 Lessons for Living – Tried and True Advice from the Wisest Americans*. Hudson Street Press, NY

Ratey, J. 2008. *Spark: The Revolutionary Science of Exercise and the Brain*. Little Brown, New York.

Rath, T. 2013. *Eat, Move, Sleep – How Small Choices Lead to Big Changes*. Missionday.

Rowe, J. W. and R. L. Kahn. *Successful Aging*. Pantheon Books, New York.

Seligman, M. E. P. 2006. *Learned Optimism: How to Change Your Mind and Your Life*. Random House, New York.

Acknowledgments

This book reflects the scientific work of thousands of people, mainly academic researchers. I am particularly indebted for the ideas I acquired from (in alphabetical order) Jonny Bowden, Edward Deci, Carol Dweck, James Fries, Eric Kim, Harold Koenig, David Kolb, Ellen Langer, Richard Lieder, Laura Putnam, Richard Ryan, Martin Seligman, David Snowden, Gary Taubes, George Vaillant, and Water Willett.

The editorial work of Jody Berman at Berman Editorial helped shape the book, helped me sharpen my message, and made my writing more accessible to non-science readers. I greatly appreciated Jody's ability to deliver honest feedback, such as, "This paragraph makes no sense," in a way that motivated me to keep plugging away to improve my writing. Jeanine Gastineau and Leila Bruno provided essential copy-editing. They couldn't help themselves from making other valuable suggestions to improve the book's readability. I thank Riley Carpenter for reformatting all of the literature citations into a coherent list and finding citation errors that I committed. Nick Zelinger of NZ Graphics designed the book. Thanks to Nick for the eye-catching cover and the engaging look of the book's interior.

The book also reflects ideas gleaned from conversations I've had with numerous people. While finishing Pacific Crest Trail hike in 2104, a half-dozen hikers graciously listened to me explain my nascent ideas about the benefits of making healthy choices. All of my hiker interviewees agreed that the healthy choices I proposed (initial versions of those in this book) made intuitive sense. Whether out of kindness or honesty, they all encouraged me to continue my research. Perhaps long-distance hikers realize that making healthy lifestyle choices will help them keep hiking, not to mention living better back home.

I could not have researched and written this book without the support of my wife, Betsy Neely. Her unflagging encouragement for what at times seemed like an endless journey helped keep me on track. Thank you, Betsy!

About the Author

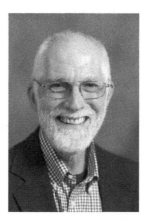

In 2013, Alan Carpenter suffered a life-threatening accident while hiking the Pacific Crest Trail in California. While incapacitated after the accident, Alan realized that he had taken his life for granted. His epiphany prompted him to learn how to recover then maintain and even increase his physical fitness, mental acuity, and spiritual grace for the rest of his life.

Over the ensuing six years, Alan combed the scientific and medical literature seeking evidence-based answers to rejuvenate his life. He synthesized what he learned into an approach to living based on nine healthy lifestyle choices that nurture body, mind, and spirit. He's also incorporated these healthy choices into his own life with outstanding results.

Since turning 61, Alan has logged 17,300 miles of long-distance hiking and cycling adventures. These include the John Muir Trail, the Colorado Trail, Pacific Crest Trail, Appalachian Trail, and 1,000 miles of the Continental Divide Trail, along with the Pacific Coast Bike Route, Southern Tier Bike Route, and Northern Tier Bike Route.

Alan has a PhD in ecology which he used in his work for The Nature Conservancy in Colorado. He founded Land Stewardship Consulting, Inc. to provide land conservation and management services to private and public clients mostly in Colorado.

Alan and his wife, Betsy Neely, have lived in Boulder for the past 30 years and have raised a daughter and a son. Alan spends his time keeping up with the latest research on health and wellness, speaking to groups, conducting workshops, and pursuing his long-distance hiking and cycling adventures.